www.wadsworth.com

wadsworth.com is the World Wide Web site for Wadsworth Publishing Company and is your direct source to dozens of online resources.

At wadsworth.com you can find out about supplements, demonstration software, and student resources. You can also send e-mail to many of our authors and preview new publications and exciting new technologies.

wadsworth.com
Changing the way the world learns®

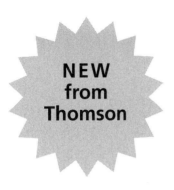

NEW from Thomson

Introduction to Careers in Health, Physical Education, and Sport

Authors: Patricia A. Floyd and Beverly J. Allen
(both of Alabama State University Montgomery, Alabama)
ISBN: 0534607853

Table of Contents

Brief Description:

This ancillary is a comprehensive guide to finding and establishing a career in the fields of Health, Physical Education and Sport. By speaking directly to the reader the book encourages students to assess and establish personal goals, develop action plans, research potential fields of employment in both the private and public sectors, create effective resumes, and suggests interviewing skills among other job searching suggestions.

The book takes them through the complicated process of picking the type of careers they want to pursue, current trends in employment, how to prepare for the transition into the working world, and insight into different types of career paths, education requirements and reasonable salary expectations. It spends time explaining the differences in credentials found in the field and testing requirements for certain professions. The authors give great advice on the best way for applicants to present themselves in a way specific to this market, which is often mistaken for being relaxed and not necessarily "professional."

There has been a special chapter added to discuss some of the legal issues that surround the workplace including discrimination and harassment. This supplement is complete with personal development activities designed to encourage the students to focus and develop better insight into their future. Helpful hints on topics such as etiquette, ethics, and legal issues as they relate to the career process, make this a tool students will keep long after they graduate.

INTRODUCTION TO PHYSICAL EDUCATION AND SPORT: FOUNDATIONS AND TRENDS

Marilyn M. Buck
Ball State University

J. Thomas Jable
William Paterson University

Patricia A. Floyd
Alabama State University

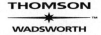
THOMSON
™
WADSWORTH

Australia • Canada • Mexico • Singapore • Spain
United Kingdom • United States

THOMSON

✦

™

WADSWORTH

Acquisitions Editor: April Lemons
Assistant Editor: Andrea Kesterke
Editorial Assistant: Madinah Chang
Technology Project Manager: Travis Metz
Marketing Manager: Jennifer Somerville
Marketing Assistant: Melanie Wagner
Advertising Project Manager: Shemika Britt
Project Manager, Editorial Production: Karen Haga
Print/Media Buyer: Barbara Britton
Permissions Editor: Elizabeth Zuber
Production Service: Robin Lockwood Productions

Text Designer: Harry Voigt
Photo Researcher: Sandra Lord
Copy Editor: Joan Pendleton
Illustrator: Ralph Lao
Cover Designer: Bill Stanton
Cover Images: Greek vase: Corbis; H.S. students: © Will McIntyre/Photo Researchers; heart monitor: © Samuel Ashfield/Getty Images
Printer: RR Donnelley
Compositor: Thompson Type

For more information about our products,
contact us at:
Thomson Learning Academic Resource Center
1-800-423-0563

For permission to use material from this text,
contact us by:
Phone: 1-800-730-2214
Fax: 1-800-730-2215
Web: http://www.thomsonrights.com

Library of Congress Control Number: 2003105865

ISBN 0-534-59850-1

Wadsworth—Thomson Learning
10 Davis Drive
Belmont, CA 94002
USA

Asia
Thomson Learning
5 Shenton Way #01-01
UIC Building
Singapore 068808

Australia/New Zealand
Thomson Learning
102 Dodds Street
Southbank, Victoria 3006
Australia

Canada
Nelson
1120 Birchmount Road
Toronto, Ontario M1K 5G4
Canada

Europe/Middle East/Africa
Thomson Learning
High Holborn House
50/51 Bedford Row
London WC1R 4LR
United Kingdom

Latin America
Thomson Learning
Seneca, 53
Colonia Polanco
11560 Mexico D.F.
Mexico

Spain/Portugal
Paraninfo
Calle/Magallanes, 25
28015 Madrid, Spain

To my students and colleagues at Ballard Junior High and Ball State University who have taught me so much.

—*Marilyn M. Buck*

To my wife, Betsy Jable, and daughter, Joy Jable, for their continuous support and encouragement during the preparation of the text.

—*J. Thomas Jable*

To Jim Thompson, a professional teacher, a dedicated coach, and a positive mentor to students.

—*Patricia A. Floyd*

About the Authors

Marilyn M. Buck, Ed.D., is a professor of Physical Education at Ball State University, Muncie, Indiana. She earned her doctorate in Physical Education from Brigham Young University (1989). Prior to obtaining the doctoral degree, Dr. Buck taught physical education and health for twelve years. She specializes in curriculum and instruction and technology in physical education. She has written another textbook and several articles and book chapters. Currently she serves as Assistant to the Chair for Sport and Physical Education. Dr. Buck has served in several leadership positions within professional organizations including President of the National Association for Physical Education in Higher Education (NAPEHE), and President of the Midwest District of the American Alliance for Health, Physical Education, Recreation, and Dance (AAHPERD). She has received the Leadership Award from the Indiana Association for Health, Physical Education, Recreation and Dance and the Service Award from NAPEHE.

J. Thomas Jable, Ph.D., M.A., M.Ed., FAAKPE is professor of Physical Education at the William Paterson University of New Jersey. He holds a Doctor of Philosophy in Physical Education (1974) with a specialization in Sport History from the Pennsylvania State University, a Master of Arts in History (1973) from Penn State and a Master of Education in Physical Education (1965) also from Penn State. In 2000 he was elected Fellow in the American Academy of Kinesiology and Physical Education. His primary teaching responsibilities include History and Philosophy of Sport and Physical Activity, Social History of Western Sport, Impact of Sport in the Modern World, and Exercise Programs for Older Adults. Since joining the faculty at William Paterson, Dr. Jable has served as chair of the Department of Exercise and Movement Sciences from 1975 to 1981 and from 1996 to 2001. Currently, he is Director of the College of Science and Health's Center for Research.

Dr. Jable is a charter member and past president of the North American Society for Sport History, serving as its president from 1985 to 1987. He also served as chair of the History of Sport and Physical Education Academy of the American Alliance for Health, Physical Education, Recreation and Dance in 1996. His research has been published in the *Journal of Sport History, The Research Quarterly of Exercise and Sport, Pennsylvania History, Pennsylvania Magazine of History and Biography, New Jersey History, The Physical Educator,* and the *Journal of Physical Education, Recreation and Dance.* Dr. Jable has also been active in the Council on Aging and Adult Development of AAHPERD where he served as the Council's first chair in 1986. He continues to serve the Council as chair of its Research Committee.

Patricia A. Floyd, Ph.D., is a professor of Physical Education at Alabama State University, Montgomery, Alabama. She holds the Doctor of Philosophy Degree in Physical Education from The Florida State University, with other degrees from The University of Alabama, Birmingham, University of Montevallo, Montevallo, Alabama, and Troy State University, Troy, Alabama. In addition to her teaching and coaching experience in grades K–12, her college and university teaching has included a wide variety of courses in physical education, health, wellness, nutrition, administration, sport, legal issues and methods, and materials courses at the elementary and high school levels.

Dr. Floyd has demonstrated professional leadership as an officer at state, district, and national levels and has made professional presentations both nationally and internationally. She has authored seven textbooks and numerous articles, and is an active writer, speaker, and consultant in the areas of wellness, health, fitness, physical education, and teacher preparation. Through these years Dr. Floyd has been active in professional and community projects, such as: organizing and sponsoring the first Jump Rope For Heart Demonstration Team in Alabama; coordinating the 1996 Alabama Olympic Celebration; serving as President of the Alabama State Association for HPERD, and the Northwest Florida Chapter of Phi Delta Kappa; organizing and developing the Pensacola Jr. College Lifestyle Improvement and Fitness Education (L.I.F.E.) Centers in Pensacola and Milton, Florida; and serving as a board member on the Alabama Governor's Commission on Physical Fitness and Sports. In addition, Dr. Floyd has received Honor Awards from Southern District, Alabama and Florida Association HPERD; American Alliance and Southern District AAHPERD Jump Rope For Heart Leadership Award; Alabama, Florida HPERD and Phi Delta Kappa, Northwest Florida Chapter Professional College Educator of the Year Awards; and the Ethnic Minority Award from Southern District and Alabama HPERD.

Contents

Preface

Physical education plays a significant role in the education of America's youth. Through physical activity, whether it be via fitness education, sport education, or mastering physical performance skills, physical education not only enhances physical attributes, but it also builds confidence and self-esteem, fosters cooperation and teamwork, promotes mutual respect, and inculcates and nourishes leadership skills. It is one of the definitive cylinders that drives the engine of education forward, contributing to the overall mission of education—nurturing youth into informed and productive adults for a democratic society.

Teaching is a noble and learned profession. As undergraduate physical education students prepare for a career in teaching, they embark on a journey that takes them through a variety of academic experiences in the sciences, social sciences, and humanities along with an immersion in pedagogical professional preparation courses. The intent of this rigorous curriculum is to prepare knowledgeable, effective, and devoted teachers who will challenge students to perform at their highest capacities.

Introduction to Physical Education and Sport: Foundations and Trends has been designed and written to inform physical education students about the profession of physical education. It gives them an orientation of the knowledge and skills physical educators must have in order to be successful in the gymnasium or classroom. It discusses the profession's heritage, including its growth and progress during the nineteenth and twentieth centuries. It analyzes philosophical constructs that assist in personalizing philosophy. It identifies critical issues facing the profession in the twenty-first century, and it projects some future directions of the profession. This text, overall, is a useful companion for students of physical education, not just for first-year undergraduates experiencing their first exposure to the profession, but also for seasoned physical education majors who will find its references, resources, Web sites, critical thinking exercises, and career guidelines helpful in upper level courses and field experiences right on through student teaching.

FEATURES

- Comprehensive coverage of the history of physical education and sport that gives students a better sense of how and why physical education and the activities related to it have developed and evolved over the years.

- Chapter 8 (Physical Education as a Profession) includes discussions on teaching Physical Education and the many careers available in physical education including discussions on "Choosing a Career," "Professional Responsibilities," and "Reasons to Teach Physical Education."

- The philosophy section in Chapter 6 includes applications to physical education, showing students the connection between theory and application.

- Each chapter includes a variety of learning tools and study references for student comprehension, including "Chapter Objectives" (5–7 bulleted objectives that describe, list, explain, define, develop, and compare chapter material) and a list of "Key Terms," which list all major key terms within each chapter, with definitions.

- "Critical Thinking Questions" appear at the end of every chapter to encourage students to review and apply the chapter material.

- End of chapter "On the Web" listings feature up to ten relevant Web sites and descriptions linked to chapter content that will expand student knowledge and understanding.

- "Multiple Choice Questions" are included at the end of each chapter and provide students with ten general questions that will help them reflect on the main topics in each chapter. Answers are provided on page 287.

- Notes and References are provided at the end of each chapter.

Ancillaries

- An Instructor's Resource CD-ROM contains helpful teaching tools as Microsoft PowerPoint slides that are linked to the chapter objectives, test questions, and the instructor's manual.

- *Introduction to Careers in Health, Physical Education, and Sport* is automatically bundled with every copy of the text. Designed to take students through the process of choosing a career and how to transition into the workplace, topics include Choosing a Career, Writing a Resume, Legal Issues, and Personal Development Activities to encourage students to focus and develop better insight into their futures.

Acknowledgments

Our thanks are gratefully extended to the publisher's reviewers and other colleagues for their insightful comments and valuable suggestions in developing this text. They include the following: Scott Colclough, Middle Tennessee State University; Dale DeVoe, Colorado State University; Peter Hastie, Auburn University; John M. Kras, Utah State University; Paulette W. Johnson, Virginia State University; Jonathan E. Nelson, Northern Michigan University; Don Rainey, Southwest Texas State University; and Cynthia D. Williams, Winston-Salem State University.

We also wish to thank Beverly Allen, Ronnie Floyd, Charlie Gibbons, Richard Morel, W. J. Parker, Glenn Rose, Jean Thompson, and Barbara Williams for their comments and assistance.

Further, we wish to thank our editor, April Lemons and the outstanding professionals at Wadsworth Publishing Company. It has been our pleasure to be associated with each of them. Their professional expertise and guidance were priceless in completing this text.

1

PHYSICAL EDUCATION: ITS NATURE AND MEANING

Chapter Objectives

After reading this chapter, the student will be able to

- Define *physical education*
- Trace the evolution of the term *physical education*
- Discuss the difference between a discipline and a profession
- Discuss how the emergence of subdisciplines changed physical education
- Explain the relationship of physical education to sport, athletics, and exercise
- Identify three major objectives of physical education
- Discuss the role of physical education in the maintenance of wellness
- Review recent developments in the promotion of physical education in schools

Physical education is a dynamic and electrifying field. It's action! It's motion! It's movement! As human beings, we are cradled in movement from womb to grave; movement insures our survival, makes us independent, and contributes to our overall health and well-being. Movement is essential in virtually every stage of our lives. Watching a toddler progress from standing to walking to running, we cheer each new motor achievement as the child grasps control of the body. We tend to sympathize with the adolescent whose uneven growth spurts create awkward movements with embarrassing outcomes. In a like manner, we empathize with a declining grandparent who needs assistance descending a staircase. In each of those examples, physical education can play a huge and decisive role. Through **fitness education,** motor development and control, physical performance competencies, and lifetime sporting activities, physical education not only improves one's quality of life but also puts life into one's years.

PHYSICAL EDUCATION: ITS MEANING AND FUNCTION

The *American Heritage Dictionary* (1996) defines physical education as "education in the care and development of the human body, stressing athletics and including hygiene."[1] *The Random House Unabridged Dictionary* (1993) regards physical education as "systematic instruction in sports, exercise, and hygiene given as part of a school or college program."[2] Though each definition is partially correct, neither one covers the true breadth and depth of the complex field of physical education. Its complexity arises out of its function as both a discipline and a profession.

The **discipline** is the body of knowledge that constitutes physical education. It is the substance or subject matter that practitioners use in applied settings. Researchers constantly study the body of knowledge and carry out experiments to discover new information about the human body and how it responds to and benefits from exercise and movement. They also search for effective ways of translating and transmitting their findings to practitioners and the public. The discipline develops a vehicle, generally a self-perpetuating

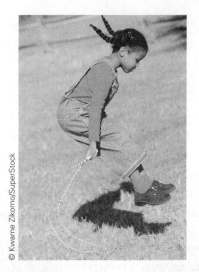

© Kwame Zikomo/SuperStock

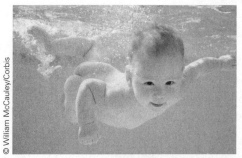

© William McCauley/Corbis

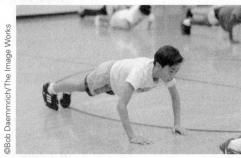

©Bob Daemmrich/The Image Works

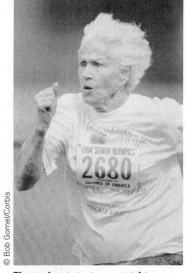

© Bob Gomel/Corbis

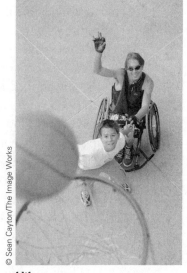

© Sean Cayton/The Image Works

Physical activity is essential in every stage of life.

organization with structure and an outlet (journal, newsletter, Web site) for disseminating information, sharing ideas, and debating issues.

The **profession** consists of practitioners (teachers, fitness/wellness instructors, and others) who apply tenets and principles of physical education in practical settings (schools, public and private agencies, clinical environments). Practitioners teach learners motor skills that contribute to efficient movement, physical fitness components that contribute to total **wellness,** and sports skills that enable the pursuit of leisure activities throughout adulthood.

THE MULTIDIMENSIONAL NATURE OF PHYSICAL EDUCATION

Physical education is as encompassing as it is unique. In carving out its own identity, physical education draws from an array of disciplines. Interwoven in its fabric are elements from the sciences, humanities, and arts. From the sciences, physical education draws heavily upon anatomy and physiology, but its connection to physics and chemistry is important for movement and nutritional analyses. Anatomy and physiology form the bulwark of physical education, serving as our basis for understanding the physiological function and anatomical structure necessary for performing athletic skills, partaking in fitness education programs, or engaging in expressive movement activities and dance forms. In striving to help people maintain optimal health through fitness, physical education teaches proper and safe techniques for carrying out health-related fitness goals—cardiovascular training, strength development, endurance training, flexibility, and body composition. Physical education also enhances the development of skill-related fitness components—power, speed, agility, balance, coordination, and reaction time. These components are instrumental for performing sports skills necessary for such activities as tennis, golf, bowling, volleyball, or softball—activities in which Americans tend to participate throughout their adult years.

Though physical education is steeped in science and medicine (preventive and hygienic), the disciplines of his-

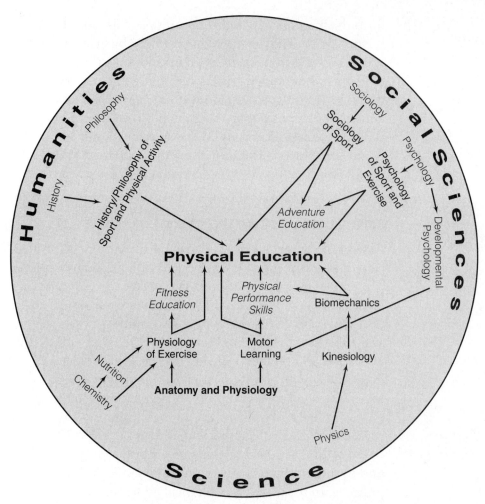

Figure 1.1 The multidimensional nature and complexity of physical education.

tory, philosophy, sociology, and psychology have played prominent roles in defining the nature of physical education. History unravels trends and courses of action physical education has followed over time. It identifies our heritage and heroes and presents significant issues and their impact on the profession. History offers remedies for problems and failures of the past and gives the discipline a sense of tradition. Philosophy helps us to develop a credo about ourselves, our ideas, our goals, and our discipline. It enables us to function within our profession and gives us direction for pursuing personal and professional goals. Social sciences—sociology and psychology—enable us to analyze group and individual actions and responses within physical education. Psychology can assist with the understanding of group or team dynamics, motivation, aggression, anxiety, and other attributes that affect the performance of physical skills, while sociology is useful for studying larger social issues involving gender and ethnicity in sport and in the profession.

EMERGENCE OF SUBDISCIPLINES

During the latter third of the twentieth century, the profession of physical education struggled with an identity crisis. The infusion of information from the sciences (physiology, kinesiology, and biomechanics) and the explosion of subdisciplines (sport history, sport philosophy, sport sociology, and sport psychology) have expanded the scope of physical education and blurred its focus. Exercise physiologists, bred traditionally in physical education departments, found they had more in common with scholars in the sciences and medicine than with their colleagues who prepare physical education teachers and athletic coaches. They opted to present their research at scientific conferences and to submit their manuscripts to scientific and medical journals. In a like manner, physical educators interested in history, philosophy, sociology, or psychology began to identify with those respective disciplines and formed organizations that reflected their academic interests. Consequently, confusion reigned. Physical educators questioned who they were and what they did. In their search for identity, physical education faculties across the country changed the names of their departments to be more representative of the way they viewed their academic orientation and degree programs. Titles such as exercise science, sport science, movement science, human movement, human performance, human kinetics, kinesiology, and kinanthropology have come to replace "physical education" in college and university departments during the past two decades. In fact, more than a hundred different names were adopted by departments that formerly contained "physical education" in their titles.[3]

More recently, **kinesiology** has become the term of choice for replacing "physical education" in departmental titles. Its broad meaning, "the study of movement," makes it a good fit for most departments offering programs in physical education, physical fitness, sports medicine, sports studies, and other areas of study in the arts, humanities, and sciences that involve physical activity. The American Academy of Kinesiology and Physical Education describes kinesiology as "a multifaceted field of study in which movement or physical activity is the intellectual focus." According to this definition, "physical activity includes exercise for improvement of health and physical fitness, activities of daily living, work, sport, dance, and play, and involves special population groups such as children and the elderly; persons with disability, injury or disease; and athletes."[4] *Kinesiology,* the primary term for the intellectual analysis of movement and physical activity, emerged from within the discipline of physical education, which itself evolved during the nineteenth century.

HISTORICAL DEVELOPMENT OF "PHYSICAL EDUCATION"

The earliest use of the term *physical education* dates back to an 1801 work by A. F. M. Willich, who defined the term as "bodily treatment of children; the term *physical* being applied in opposition to moral."[5] Right from the beginning, "physical education" carried a moral connotation. A quarter of a century later, the *American Journal of Education* and the *Boston Medical Intelligencer* elevated the visibility of physical education by reinforcing its moral implications and giving it an educational component when both journals requested schools to establish "corporeal exercise" programs consisting of "healthful exercise and innocent recreations."[6] During the 1830s, Charles Caldwell, John C. Warren, and Andrew Combe, all physicians, extolled the benefits of physical education. But to them, physical education was more than mere "bodily education." It was a much broader term that encompassed the mental and moral aspects of human nature as well—thereby serving as the basis of humankind's quest for perfectibility.[7]

Also during the 1830s, but perhaps even earlier, the term *physical culture* came into vogue in America. It, too, initially had moral implications as John Jeffries' 1833 article, "Physical Culture, the Result of Moral Obligation" revealed in discussing the relationship of body and soul.[8] But by the end of the century, the meaning of *physical culture* was different from that of *physical education*. The former term dealt with the development of the body by exercise, while the latter consisted of instruction in bodily exercises and games, especially in schools. A third popular term, *physical training*, distinct from the other two, meant the systematic use of exercises to promote physical fitness.[9] In school settings, physical education incorporated elements of sport, athletics, and exercise to reach its goals.

THE RELATIONSHIP OF PHYSICAL EDUCATION TO SPORT, ATHLETICS, AND EXERCISE

Since its inception and recognition as a field of study, physical education has embraced—and still does—a variety of exercise to strengthen and condition the human body. Then, when sports and games were introduced into the curriculum during the early twentieth century, sports performance skills received considerable emphasis. Those skills were used in contests held during physical education classes and in interschool athletic competitions. Although athletics, by their extracurricular nature, lie outside the purview of physical education, both athletics and physical education can offer valuable lessons for each other. Sports performance skills can be taught and developed in physical education classes, and athletic principles can be applied in physical education classes to provide experiences dealing with the nature of competition, the necessity of teamwork, the joy of success, and the management of failure—all of which are part of life. In addition to its connection with sports and athletics, physical education has had a close alliance with health, recreation, and dance.

THE ALLIANCE WITH HEALTH, RECREATION, AND DANCE

Fitness and wellness (that is, total well-being) goals pull physical education and health together for common

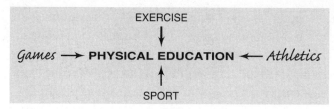

Figure 1.2 Sport, athletics, games, and exercise are all connected to physical education.

purposes. Although physical education is an outgrowth of nineteenth-century health reform (as discussed in Chapter 4), it emerged as a discipline with its own identity in the late nineteenth century. But with compatible goals, it was only natural for health and physical education to build an alliance, and they did so in 1937 when the American Physical Education Association merged with the Department of School Health and Physical Education of the National Education Association to form the American Association of Health and Physical Education (AAHPE).

Recreation, valuable for providing effective outlets for leisure, often as physical activity, was a natural ally of health and physical education. It joined AAHPE in 1938 to create AAHPER. Then, dance, with its expressive movement and art forms, allied with the other disciplines in 1979. Thus the American Alliance for Health, Physical Education, Recreation and Dance (AAHPERD) represents the connections among these four disciplines and disseminates information about them through its public information channels, professional journals, and news organs.

The discipline begets the profession and the profession opens doors for career opportunities. The topic of careers will be discussed more thoroughly in Chapter 10, but some of the professional opportunities emanating from physical education and its allied disciplines are found in teaching, coaching, health promotion, fitness and wellness programs, research, rehabilitation and sports medicine, and athletic and sports administration.

CONTEMPORARY TRENDS AND ISSUES

The U.S. Department of Education reported that the country will need more than one million new teachers by 2010,[10] and a sizeable number will be needed to fill vacancies in physical education. In spite of those projections, physical education programs face the constant threat of reduction, if not total elimination, due to budget constraints and poor student performance in mathematics, science, and English. The adoption of core-content **standards** and curricula assessments by most states have placed added pressure on school districts to improve student performance in classroom subjects, oftentimes at the expense of physical education. The *2001 Shape of the Nation Report* conducted by the National Association of Sport and Physical Education (NASPE) revealed that Illinois was the only state that requires daily physical education for all students, K–12, while Alabama requires daily physical education for all K–8 pupils. Two states, Colorado and South Dakota, do not have any mandate for physical education. Although most states have some type of legislative mandate calling for physical education, they allow local school districts to determine time allotment and curricular content.[11]

Even more discouraging were the results of the Centers for Disease Control and Prevention's (CDC) *School Health Policies and Programs Study (SHPPS)* released in 2001. It revealed that 8.0 percent of the elementary schools, 6.4 percent of the middle/junior high schools, and 5.8 percent of the senior high schools across the United States provided daily physical education for students at all grade levels during an entire school year.[12]

Compulsory physical education has declined in spite of overwhelming evidence proclaiming the importance and necessity of physical activity for people of all ages. *Physical Activity and Health: A Report of the Surgeon General* (1996) presents a clear message that even moderate amounts of daily physical activity can enhance quality of life and improve health. Even more emphatically, the report states that "physical activity reduces the risk of premature mortality in general, and of coronary heart disease, hypertension, colon cancer, and diabetes mellitus in particular. Physical activity also improves mental health and is important for the health of muscles, bones, and joints."[13] *Healthy People 2010* (2000) concurs with the findings of the *Surgeon General's Report,* for its major physical activity goal for 2010 is to "improve health, fitness, and quality of life through daily physical activity." Because only one of thirteen physical activity and fitness objectives of *Healthy People 2000* was met for the year 2000, the 2010 objectives call for 30 percent of adults (eighteen years and older) and 35 percent of children and adolescents to engage in moderate physical activity.[14]

Reaching this objective will be one of America's great challenges at a time when the incidence of overweight and obesity continues to climb among its youth. The recently released *Surgeon General's Call to Action to Prevent and Decrease Overweight and Obesity* disclosed that 13 percent of children (ages six to fourteen) and 14 percent of adolescents (ages twelve to nineteen) are overweight, a trend that has increased threefold for adolescents over the past two decades. Directly related to overweight conditions in youth are an increase in risk factors for heart disease; hypertension and elevated cholesterol levels; type 2 diabetes, which generally affects adults; and social discrimination due to excess weight, which often leads to poor self-esteem. Evidence for overweight conditions points to lack of physical activity and poor diet, or a combination of the two, though genetics, lifestyle, and environment have some influence as well. The prime culprits are television and computer and video games, as 43 percent of adolescents watch more than two hours of television each day.[15]

The future, however, is not bleak. Educators and government agencies are already laying the foundation to promote physical activity. *Healthy People 2010* established ten high-priority public health areas, with physical activity to be the first leading health indicator. The report declares physical education as the "primary source of physical activity and fitness instruction" for children and adolescents. Its objectives, therefore, recommend increasing the proportion of schools that require daily physical education, increasing the proportion of adolescents who participate in daily physical education, and increasing the percentage of physical education class time in which students are physically active.[16] In November 2000, at the request of President Clinton, the Secretary of Health and Human Services and the Secretary of Education released their joint report, *Promoting Better Health for Young People through Physical Activity and Sports,* which called for the "renewal of physical education in our schools and the expansion of after-school programs that offer physical activity and sports."[17] One month later, the U.S. Congress passed the Physical Education for Progress (PEP) Act, which made $400 million available over five years to increase physical education in the schools. The initial $5 million appropriation for 2001 has been made available in the form of grants to local school districts. Congress authorized and appropriated another $50 million for the 2002 fiscal year. But each year Congress must authorize a specific appropriation for the PEP grants, so it is not known whether the remaining $345 million will be available in future years.[18]

Recently, NASPE asked a group of physical education professionals to develop a working definition of a physically educated person. After developing the definition, the group created benchmarks for grades K, 2, 4, 6, 8, 10, and 12 that illustrate progress expected in a high-quality daily physical education program. The next phase consisted of writing national standards for physical education, which was part of the movement to develop national and state standards in all subject fields. All of those developments are positive signs for the field of physical education as we enter the twenty-first century.

PHYSICAL EDUCATION: A DEFINITIONAL APPROACH

Physical education, as this chapter has shown, is a complex term. In its strictest sense, it is formal instruction in the care, development, and improvement of one's physical capacities. More broadly, however, it connects with intellectual, social, and emotional, as well as physical, components of *wellness,* our modern-day conception of optimal health and total well-being. Physical education activities can reduce stress by decreasing muscle tension, foster social relationships by encouraging group participation, and stimulate cognitive function by providing experiences that increase blood flow and hormone secretions in the brain.

Physical education's most obvious connection to the wellness framework falls within its physical dimension, which is apparent in its goals. Traditionally, physical education goals have been classified into three domains—psychomotor, cognitive, and affective. **Psychomotor goals** establish competence levels for executing physical performance skills, physical fitness, and lifetime physical activities. The **cognitive goals** invoke learning experiences that nurture self-expression, problem solving, and socialization, while **affective goals** inculcate habits and attitudes that reinforce participation in physical activity, enhance feelings of well-being, and cultivate self-esteem.

Because physical education draws upon elements from wellness, health, exercise, sports, athletics, recreation, and other related areas, it can be defined as a process that uses physical activity to develop and enrich one's physical, cognitive, social, and emotional faculties for the purpose of enhancing one's quest for total well-being.

On the Web

www.aahperd.org/naspe
Official Web page of National Association of Sport & Physical Education, an association of the American Alliance for Health, Physical Education, Recreation and Dance. Information is available about reports, publications, and conferences.

www.cdc.gov/publications.htm
Web page of the Centers for Disease Control and Prevention. Contains reports and executive summaries of reports. Includes link to *U.S. Surgeon General's Report on Physical Activity and Health and Healthy People 2010*. Lists CDC's other publications, software, and other products.

http://edStandards.org/Standards.html
Contains educational standards and assessments by subject and by state.

http://ericeece.org/statlink.html
Provides links to each state's Department of Education.

http://www.pelinks4u.org/links/advocacy.htm
Provides links to resources for physical education advocacy efforts.

Key Terms

affective goals Physical education objectives that promote an appreciation for and positive attitude toward physical activity through pleasurable and meaningful experiences (page 13).

cognitive goals Physical education objectives that advocate challenging physical activities involving problem solving, cooperative ventures, or individual self-expression to stimulate thought processes (page 13).

discipline The body of knowledge that constitutes physical education (page 2).

fitness education Process of developing and improving health-related fitness components (cardiovascular endurance, muscular strength, muscular endurance, flexibility, and body composition) (page 2).

kinesiology A multifaceted field of study in which movement or physical activity is the intellectual focus (page 7).

profession Field in which one practices one's vocation (page 4).

psychomotor goals Physical education objectives that emphasize performance competencies (page 13).

standards Prescribed levels of performance that indicate what students should know and what they should be able to do (page 10).

wellness Optimal health and total well-being, generally involving physical, intellectual, social, emotional, and spiritual dimensions (page 4).

Multiple Choice Questions

1. The term for the body of knowledge that constitutes physical education is
   a. profession
   b. discipline
   c. standard
   d. humanities

2. What is the bulwark of physical education?
   a. sport sociology and sport psychology
   b. sports and athletics
   c. teaching and coaching
   d. anatomy and physiology

3. The first addition to the American Physical Education Association was
   a. health
   b. recreation
   c. sport
   d. dance

4. The decrease in physical education requirements is due to all but one of the following:

   a. budget shortfalls
   b. comparison of student performance in physical education with performance in other subjects
   c. development of state standards and graduation assessments
   d. joint resolution in both houses of U.S. Congress

5. The first leading health indicator of the CDC's *Healthy People 2010 Report* is

   a. tobacco usage
   b. nutrition
   c. physical activity
   d. obesity

6. The joint congressional resolution that authorizes $400 million over the next five years to increase physical education in the schools is

   a. the Physical Education for Progress (PEP) Act
   b. The Surgeon General's report on physical activity and health
   c. *Healthy People 2010*
   d. *School Health Policies and Practices Survey* (*SHPPS* 2000)

7. In the past thirty years, obesity among American school age children has

   a. remained the same
   b. doubled
   c. tripled
   d. quadrupled

8. Which one of the following is *not* a domain for physical education goals?

   a. psychomotor
   b. cognitive
   c. affective
   d. creative

9. An increasingly popular term for replacing *physical education* in department titles is

   a. anthropology
   b. kinanthropology
   c. kinesiology
   d. kinesthetics

10. The earliest known use of the term *physical education* dates back to

    a. 1601
    b. 1701
    c. 1801
    d. 1901

Critical Thinking Questions

1. Discuss the difference between a discipline and a profession.

2. Explain how the emergence of subdisciplines in physical education has changed the field.

3. Describe the relationship of physical education to sport, athletics, and exercise.

4. Define *wellness* and explain how physical education can contribute to it.

5. Identify at least three reports that advocate increasing physical education participation among schoolchildren. Then discuss their major recommendations.

Notes and References

1. *American Heritage Dictionary of the English Language*, 3d ed.

2. *Random House Unabridged Dictionary*, 2d ed.

3. S. E. Brassie and J. E. Razor, "HPER Unite Names in Higher Education—A View Towards the Future," *JOPERD*, 60, No. 7 (1989): 33–40.

4. American Academy of Kinesiology and Physical Education Web site, www.aakpe.org

5. Quoted in Jack W. Berryman, "Exercise and Medical Tradition from Hippocrates through Antebellum America: A Review Essay," in *Sport and Exercise Sciences: Essays in the History of Sports Medicine*, ed. Jack W. Berryman and Roberta J. Park (Urbana: University of Illinois Press, 1992), 43.

6. Quoted in Roberta J. Park, "Physiologists, Physicians, and Physical Educators: Nineteenth-Century Biology and Exercise, *Hygienic* and *Educative*," *Journal of Sport History*, 14, no. 1 (Spring 1987): 37.

7. Berryman, 43–44; Roberta J. Park, "Health, Exercise, and the Biomedical Impulse," *Research Quarterly for Exercise and Sport*, 61, no. 2 (June 1990): 128.

8. Park, 128.

9. *Oxford English Dictionary*.

10. Barbara Kantrowitz and Pat Wingert, "Who Will Teach Our Kids," *Newsweek*, 2 October 2000, 37–42.

11. National Association for Sport and Physical Education, *2001 Shape of the Nation Report: Status of Physical Education in the USA* (Reston, Va.: American Alliance for Health, Physical Education, Recreation and Dance, 2001), 3.

12. School Health Policies and Programs Study (SHPPS 2000), Fact Sheet, Physical Education and Activity, Centers for Disease Control and

Prevention (CDC) Web site, www.cdc.gov/nccdphp/dash/factsheets/
fs00_pe.htm.

13. U.S. Department of Health and Human Services, *Physical Activity and
Health: A Report of the Surgeon General* (Atlanta: Centers for Disease Control and Prevention, National Center for Chronic Disease Prevention
and Health Promotion, 1996), 4.

14. *Healthy People 2010, Understanding and Improving Health,* CDC Web
site, http://web/health.gov/healthypeople/Document/HTML/Volume2/
22Physical.htm, 5.

15. U.S. Department of Health and Human Services, *The Surgeon
General's Call to Action to Prevent and Decrease Overweight and Obesity*
(Rockville, Md.: Public Health Service, Office of the Surgeon General,
2001), Section 1.2, 1–2; Section 1.4, 1.

16. *Healthy People 2010,* 34.

17. National Center for Chronic Disease Prevention and Health Promotion, *Chronic Disease Notes & Reports,* 14, no. 1 (Winter 2001): 10–13.

18. National Association for Physical Education & Sport Web site,
www.aahperd.org/naspe

2

LIFE, SPORT, AND SPECTACLE IN ANCIENT SOCIETIES

Chapter Objectives

After reading this chapter, the student will be able to

- Describe the relationships between sport and survival, ritual, and adventure

- Identify at least two sporting activities related to survival in China, India, Mesopotamia, Egypt, and sub-Saharan Africa

- Define *arête*

- Compare the educational practices of Sparta with those of ancient Athens

- Identify and describe at least three events held at the ancient Olympic games

- Identify at least four spectacles that were held in ancient Rome

- Explain the motives of emperors and political aspirants for sponsoring games

Physical activity is inherent to human life. It is essential for the health and well-being of the body. From the beginning of recorded history and even during the preliterate era, physical activity has taken a variety of forms—play, sport, athletic competition, exercise, recreation—depending on the culture and its nature and orientation. Some cultures may have only the play element, while others, like modern America, have all of those forms. The meaning and uses of physical activity, too, vary from culture to culture. For some cultures, physical activity is an expressive art form (dance); for others, a recreational pursuit. Work, too, generally involves physical activity, though recent technological developments have reduced the need for physical labor in some sectors of the modern workplace. Some scholars consider work as the opposite of sport, a direct extension of play, while others hold that forms of work are embedded in sport, as with professional athletics. Our intent is not to delineate spheres of work and play or to draw the fine line of work within sport. We recognize the relationships of work and sport and consider these entities to be mutually beneficial. Across eons of time, however, physical activity in most cultures has been connected to survival (military preparation), ritual (religion), and/or adventure (gambling). Those trends were evident in ancient civilizations.

CHINA

In China the martial arts date back to the Zhou civilization (eleventh century to 771 B.C.E.). Early fighting skills consisted of archery, horseriding, charioteering, and wrestling. Later, with the emergence of the infantry foot soldier, running, jumping, and throwing became important training vehicles. As Chinese society changed with each dynasty, so too did its military training and techniques. By the time of the Han dynasty (206 B.C.E. to 24 C.E.), riding skills had replaced charioteering; wrestling had adopted more sophisticated maneuvers; archery skills improved considerably due to more intensive training; bare-handed fighting, along with kicking and striking skills, appeared on the scene; and fencing and swordplay received increasingly more attention.

Sporting and recreational activities reinforced the martial skills necessary for survival and protection. Other activities derived from military training were tug-of-war, football (soccer), weight lifting, polo, hurdles, jumping, and boxing. Outside of military training, there was no competition in Chinese sport. The Chinese were more interested in morality, ethics, and character development, and their physical activities, for the most part, reflected these interests.

Not all of China's physical activities were oriented toward the military. There is evidence of religious-philosophical connections. Shakyamuni, founder of Buddhism, was fond of sport, and mural scenes of his youth depict horse riding, wrestling, archery, swimming, and boating. In later periods Buddhist monks, trained in kung fu and weapons, repelled invaders during the Manchu dynasty with aspirations of restoring the Ming dynasty.

Surprisingly, there is considerable evidence of Chinese women's involvement in sport. Women were known to swim, boat, fish, throw balls, shoot archery, fly kites, and play polo, football, and golf.[1]

INDIA

In India the Hindu lifestyle subjugated material pleasures to spiritual salvation. As a consequence, physical activity and exercise had little value among Hindus, who promoted a life of asceticism and spiritual cleansing that ran the gamut from moderation to self-inflicted torture. Moreover, their nonviolent approach to hostility reinforced the futility of survival skills training and physical conditioning except for the military caste, which engaged in spear and javelin throwing; sword, sling, and battle-axe play; and archery. During peacetime, the military caste hunted in order to keep battle skills sharp.

Buddhism came to India during the third century B.C.E. as a reaction to the austerity of Hinduism. Buddhists viewed exercise as an important component of health and an acceptable recreational outlet. They did, however, attempt to suppress the gambling and dice games that were common in

India. They were also alarmed at the betting that took place on bull, cock, elephant, ram, and rhinoceros fights. Polo, wrestling, and dance existed in India, but its hallmark activity was **yoga.** Indians believed that physical strength and stamina were essential for meditation and the spiritual cleansing that occurred with yoga.[2]

MESOPOTAMIA

In ancient times, Sumerians inhabited the area in the Tigris and Euphrates River valleys (present-day Iraq). They constructed cities, devised and promulgated laws to regulate behavior, and developed cuneiform writing, which enabled the recording and expression of ideas. Sumerians were hunters and warriors who mastered the chariot and the combat sports of boxing and wrestling. They also participated in archery, running, and swimming to maintain physical stamina and proficiency with weapons for warfare.[3]

EGYPT

As in Mesopotamia, hunting was a popular activity in Egypt and a privilege of aristocrats. Egyptians hunted lions, hippopotami, wild bulls, and just about any other animal found in the Nile Valley. The hunters' chief weapon was the bow and arrow, although for some hunts, they speared fish or killed birds with a stick. In addition to providing recreation for the Egyptians, hunting kept their military skills sharp. Effective warriors, Egyptians also practiced target archery and used the chariot and horse successfully in battle. Wrestling, as in other cultures, was paramount. The Egyptians engaged in stick fighting, but, surprisingly, did not emphasize boxing. The Nile River made boating, rowing, swimming, and fishing attractive. People engaged in competitive ball games, children's games, and board games. Acrobatics and dance provided entertainment, but those activities also had religious connections to Egyptian gods.

The connection of sport to ritual and gaming in Egyptian society can be seen in the **Festival of Sed** and the Senet board game. During the Festival of Sed, Egyptian rulers ran a course consisting of semicircular tracks to demonstrate their physical prowess and to reaffirm control over their subjects. Pharaohs periodically repeated this ritual during their reign, symbolically, renewing their strength and magical powers. Furthermore, semicircular tracks were normally built near tombs so deceased monarchs could undertake this ritual of renewal in the hereafter. The Senet board game was the Egyptians' favorite. It contained elements of chance and guessing as contestants sought to move objects toward their objectives. In some versions, the course that one selected symbolized pathways on which the dead traveled to reach their final resting place in the next world.[4]

SUB-SAHARAN AFRICA

As in other early cultures, people south of the Sahara participated in physical activities that developed and maintained their survival and martial skills. Wrestling was a universal practice in this part of Africa, though not necessarily a universal medium for military preparation. In some areas it was recreational and ceremonial, for it was sometimes accompanied by music, songs, dance, and magic. One could hardly distinguish between recreation and serious ceremony. In some locales, wrestling also served as a rite of passage for both boys and girls. Stick fighting schooled youth in elements of self-defense. Ball playing, target games, top spinning, foot races, jumping contests, and swimming were also common among boys and men. Although few girls and women took up swimming, most participated in dance.

For sub-Saharan Africans, dance was an expressive art form with recreational, ceremonial, and ritualistic meanings. The nature and vigor of even recreational dance routines contributed to the physical condition of male and female participants. In performing warrior dances, men invoked divine intervention to bring them success in battle. Both men and women danced at religious festivals and ceremonies.

Gaming and adventure activities were evident throughout the sub-Saharan region. The most common board game, *mancalo,* involved placing objects (stones, nuts, seeds, or beans) in strategic positions with the intent of capturing the opponents' objects. This game of capture relies on judicious calculation mingled with elements of chance.[5]

EDUCATION AND GYMNASTICS IN ANCIENT GREECE

Ancient Greece consisted of a collection of cities (or city-states), each with its own political autonomy and economic independence. From time to time, though, certain cities formed alliances for protection against invaders or for economic benefits. Pervading Greek culture was the ideological concept of **arête,** in which Greeks strove for excellence in all areas: physically, intellectually, and spiritually. Though few Greeks, or people of any culture for that matter, could reach this pinnacle, excellence remained their goal. It gave them purpose and direction and influenced their lifestyles. Sparta and Athens, two of the dominant and most heralded cities of ancient Greece, pursued excellence in different ways—with disparate lifestyles, educational systems, and physical training pursuits.

Sparta was one of the first utopian or communal states. Although Spartans initially subscribed to *arête,* they abandoned this ideology under the leadership of Lycurgus in 650 B.C.E., when *helots,* whom they had enslaved, revolted and nearly overthrew them. From that time onward, Spartans emphasized military training and focused on physical fitness and obedience to authority. Both boys and girls received vigorous training and participated in dance, choral singing, and competitive athletic contests during their preadolescent years. Spartans wanted robust, physically strong men and women to produce healthy offspring. During adolescence, Spartan males were further prepped for battle through an austerity program that forced them to live on a meager diet and endure severe climatic conditions for months at a time with bare feet and scant clothing. Here, too, they learned resourcefulness. Stealing food, though innately immoral in Spartan culture, was essential for survival. If caught, however, the culprit received a double punishment—one for committing the theft and a second for getting caught. Although Spartans deserve praise for developing physical fitness, fostering courage, and promoting gender equality, they jettisoned culture (wisdom, prudence, justice, and the like) when they abandoned *arête,* leaving them with little, other than war, to enjoy. Consequently, when hostilities ceased, Spartans could not handle the luxury of peace, which contributed to their decline.

Athenians, on the other hand, continuously strove for *arête.* Their education consisted of letters, music, philosophy, law, math, and gymnastics (that is, physical education). But in Athens, only boys had these educational opportunities, for girls were restricted to domestic crafts. Boys from Athens's upper stratum received instruction at private schools. Instruction in gymnastics was generally given at a **palestra** by the *paidotribe,* or trainer. At the *palestra,* young boys learned to wrestle, box, run, jump, and throw. Because *palestras* were generally small, instruction and practice in throwing and running events often occurred at the more elaborate **gymnasia,** which, for the most part, were public institutions. At age eighteen, all Athenian young men underwent two years of military training, mandated by the city-state. Gymnastics was essential preparation for this stage. Military preparedness was just as important to Athenians as it was to Spartans, but Athenians had a much broader conception of life and a wider view of education, for they insisted on the development of character and taste, in conjunction with harmonious development of the body, mind, and spirit.

GREEK ATHLETICS AND THE OLYMPIC GAMES

For the ancient Greeks, athletic contests had meaning in terms of religious connections, military readiness, and aesthetic appreciation. Whether reflected in the sculpture of Myron's discus thrower or nudity in the athletic arena, the Greeks admired the body for its symmetrical development. The ultimate expression of body symmetry is evident in the Doryphoros, by Polykleitos, who cast a young athlete, thought to be Achilles, in perfect human form.

But long before Greeks began to admire the beauty of an athlete's proportional physique, Greek athletes were

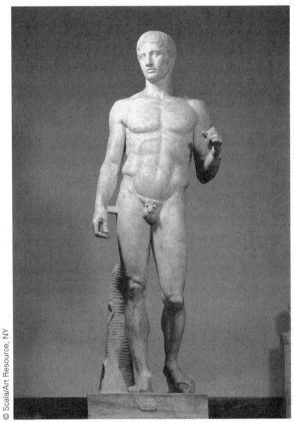

Doryphoros, the perfect athlete with the evenly proportioned symmetrical body.

steeped in ritual and religion. The earliest athletic contests were spontaneous events that grew out of funerary rites. Often games were held instantaneously on the spot to honor a fallen warrior. One classic example appears in Book XXIII of Homer's *Iliad*, when Achilles holds games to honor Patroclus, his compatriot who died in battle on the plains of Troy. Achilles organizes a series of eight events to pay homage to his deceased comrade. The ancient Greeks believed that athletic contests gave needed energy to the deceased, enabling them to make the journey to their final destination in the afterlife.[6] They also devoted athletic contests to a variety of gods whom they hoped would bestow favors upon them, such as rainfall or plentiful crops; sometimes the contests were just a demonstration of gratitude to the gods for honoring their requests. Gradually, with the passage of time, the spontaneity of athletic competition yielded to athletic contests that were held at regular intervals defined by the position of the moon.

The **Olympic Games,** dating back to 776 B.C.E. were held every forty-eight lunar months. Initially a foot race to the altar of Zeus, the Olympics expanded with events and activities over the centuries until 472 B.C.E., when they became a stabilized, five-day festival involving processions, oaths, prayers, hymns, and sacrifices to the gods along with the athletic contests.

The competition began with contests for trumpeters and heralds and contests for boys. On the second day there were chariot races, horse races, a foot race (a stade race—one length of the stadium), and the **pentathlon** (discus, javelin, jump, foot race, and wrestling). The first athlete to win three events captured the pentathlon. Next followed a day of foot races, processions, and a sacrifice to Zeus. The heavy events took place on the fourth day and included boxing (no rules, weight classes, or rounds), wrestling (in which an opponent had to be thrown to the ground), a race in armor, and *pankration*, the most brutal of all Greek athletic contests. The *pankration,* consisting of boxing, wrestling, and kicking, continued until one of the participants was driven into submission through relentless punching, kicking, and the functional scissors, which freed one's hands for the lethal choke hold. Strangely enough, biting and gouging were prohibited, but those infractions were not always enforced. Arrichion, two-time Olympic *pankration* champion, succumbed at the games of the 54th Olympiad when his opponent held him down with a scissors hold and choked him to death with his free hands.[7] The last day was reserved for the closing ceremonies and crowning of victors.

The victors were crowned with an olive wreath, which had little face value but far-reaching symbolic value. In most instances, city-states bestowed upon a victorious athlete free

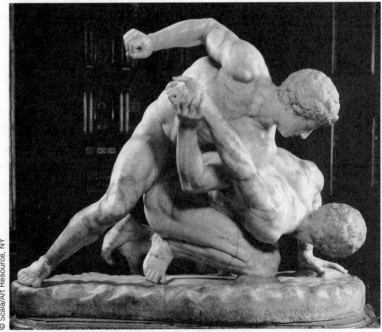

© Scala/Art Resource, NY

Pankratiasts used arm, leg, and choke holds to force their opponents into submission.

meals for life, a place of honor at public events, and other amenities. So serious about the Olympic games were the Greeks that they established an Olympic truce that enabled athletes to pass through war zones unmolested on their way to Olympia. Actually, Olympic competitors first went to Elis, a nearby training site, where they spent thirty days preparing for the games. Morality, too, played a large role at Olympia. If an athlete was caught violating the rules, he was memorialized for posterity as a cheater. His name was carved on the base of a statue, created in the image of Zeus, called a *zane.* In nearly 1,200 years of Olympic competition, only eleven zanes were erected.

The **Olympic Games** were the most prestigious but not the only Panhellenic games. The Greeks held other athletic competitions at Delphi (Pythian in honor of Apollo), Corinth (Isthmian in honor of Poseidon), and Nemea (Nemean in honor of Zeus). Known as **crown games,** these contests were held regularly during non-Olympic years. The Panhellenic stature of these games and the benefits gained from victory attracted athletes from all over the Greek world—just as the Olympics did. While aristocratic athletes had the financial resources to travel to and compete in crown games, athletes of low birth had to parlay their earnings from victories at local festivals into a chance at the highly valued prizes of Panhellenic competition.

The **Panathenaic Festival,** one of the most prominent local competitions, offered some of the most lucrative prizes. Classicist David Young has calculated the value of winning the Panathenaic stade race at 1,200 drachmas (100 amphorae of olive oil at 12 drachmas each). This equates to 847 days' wages or nearly three years of work. The purchasing power of 1,200 drachmas in ancient Greece could bring six or seven slaves, 100 sheep, or two or three homes. Thus, a successful athlete could lead a comfortable life. A single victory at Athens could earn a competitor more in a few seconds than he could earn laboring for an entire year.[8]

Greek athletics waned and declined as Roman influences began to infiltrate Greece during the second century B.C.E. The death knell tolled for the Olympics in 394 C.E. after the Emperor Theodosius adopted Christianity and banned the games for their idolatrous connections to pagan gods. Then, too, Greek athletes themselves contributed to their downfall when they abandoned the concept of **arête.** They adopted a meat diet over grain in order to bulk up for the heavy events that did not have weight classes and in so doing lost the proportional development of the body. Upper body girth and strength replaced body symmetry. Though professionalism had been present in Greek athletics early on (witness five-time Olympic wrestling champion Milo of Croton, sixth century B.C.E.; Theogenes, boxing and *pankration* victor in the fifth century B.C.E.), in later years mercenaries in the form of pot hunters and tramp athletes eagerly traveled from games to games in search of victory and its accompanying spoils. Competition among city-states for champion athletes to represent them at various crown games was also a factor in the deterioration of Greek athletics. Croton, a city in a Greek colony on the Italian peninsula, recruited athletes and rewarded their success, probably with monies from its treasury. Croton's athletes won 23 of 109 Olympic events from 588 to 484 B.C.E. No other Crotonian won at Olympia after 484 B.C.E., but some of Croton's stellar athletes competed for other city-states, like Syracuse. The combination of all of these forces diminished the stature of athletic competition and ultimately led to the downfall of Greek athletics.[9]

THE FEMALE IN GREEK SPORT

While men competed in the Olympics and other crown games, women in ancient Greece had little opportunity to participate in sporting activities. In Athens and most Greek city-states, women were schooled in domestic crafts and, for the most part, were semisecluded. The exception, of course, was Sparta, where women participated vigorously in athletic contests until they reached childbearing age. The intent there was to develop strong, healthy women for the production of healthy offspring. Spartan women, like their male counterparts, competed in the nude. This erotic feature encouraged matrimony and gave men an opportunity to view and select future brides.

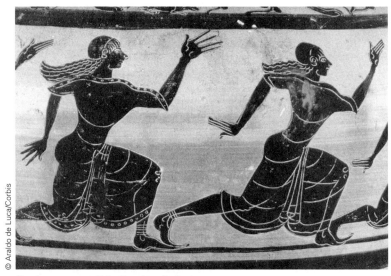

© Araldo de Luca/Corbis

Greek women participating in a foot race.

Women did compete in games devoted to the goddess Hera, known as the **Heraia,** which were held at Olympia a month before Olympic competition. These were prenuptial rites of passage in which adolescent girls made the transition to the childbearing years. This competition served also as a fertility rite. Archeological evidence uncovered at Brauron near Athens revealed that some Athenian maidens wore bear masks as they participated in dances and races devoted to Artemis, goddess of purity and procreation. The bear mask ritual symbolized "the girls' transition from savagery (as 'bears') to civilization."

Greek annals portray Atalanta as a runner, wrestler, and huntress. Legend has it that this great runner, who could outrun men as well as women, was not interested in marriage, but agreed to marry the first man who could outrun her. She defeated a number of suitors, but fell victim to Melanion, who, assisted by the chicanery of Aphrodite, distracted Atalanta by tossing golden apples in her path. As she paused to examine the apples, Melanion beat her to the finish line and took her as his bride.

As a female, Atalanta never had the opportunity to participate in the Olympic Games, nor did any other Greek female, for that matter. Kynisca, a Spartan princess, received the olive wreath at Olympia as a surrogate participant in the early fourth century B.C.E. when her horses won the chariot race. In the ancient games, the horses' owner, not the charioteer, received the victory crown. Kynisca proclaimed herself as the only woman in the Greek world to hold the victory crown from Olympia.[11]

LIFE AND EDUCATION IN THE ROMAN WORLD

While athletics developed and the Olympic Games unfolded in ancient Greece, Romans moved to become the dominant culture on the Italian peninsula around 509 B.C.E., when they conquered the neighboring Etruscans who had settled there centuries earlier. In this process Etruscan funerary games, ceremonial sacrifices, and gladiatorial duels found their way into Roman life. By 275 B.C.E., Rome had unified the Italian peninsula under its command and began to expand its influence as far west as Spain and east to Greece. The Roman Republic instituted a representative type of political system—actually, a senatorial republic composed of aristocrats. The Republic expanded and flourished under Julius Caesar, but ended with his death in 44 B.C.E. After a tumultuous struggle for power among Caesar's lieutenants, Augustus emerged and established the bureaucratic structure that governed and administered the vast territory that became the Roman Empire.[12]

Education in the Republic occurred in the home as the father schooled his son(s) in the Twelve Tables, a moral code of behavior. In addition to morality, Romans emphasized loyalty to the state and physical prowess necessary for a strong military. At age seventeen, aristocratic males underwent military training. As a result of Greek influence, elementary schools began to appear in the second century B.C.E. and were firmly instituted during the Empire. The curriculum consisted of reading, writing, and math, with some Latin and Greek. Secondary schools emerged, too, with oratory, debate, and philosophy receiving attention. Oratory prepared young Romans for arguing issues in the senate or commanding military units. Formal education was restricted to males; patrician females learned rhythmic movements and dance, mastered the supervision of slaves who performed domestic chores, and married at puberty. Their primary function was childbearing and child rearing. Plebeian women, on the other hand, toiled in the fields and sold their goods at the marketplace.[13]

Military training was crucial for Rome's aspirations, for newly conquered territories had to be administered and controlled. Early on, fathers took their sons to the **Campus Martius,** a type of parade-ground assembly point where youth and men sharpened their martial skills by boxing, wrestling, throwing the discus and javelin, practicing archery, and racing horses and chariots. Some youth also engaged in catch and toss and handball-like games. Though Roman lads used athletic activities chiefly as a medium for military preparedness, a small number of patrician girls and women participated for apparently personal and otherwise unde-termined reasons. They entered foot races at Rome's Capitoline Games and at the Augustalia and Sebasteia cele-brated at Naples.[14] Apart from its association with battle-field skills, athletic competition was rare in Rome because its citizenry turned to spectator activities for their entertain-ment pleasures.

ROMAN SPECTACLES

Roman spectacles consisted of festivals (*feriae*), public games (*ludi*), and shows (*munera*). Festivals initially were feasts to propitiate the gods to benefit agriculture (plentiful crops, adequate rainfall) or to eliminate pestilence (plague, disease). At festivals, religious clerics performed rites, generally in-volving ceremonial sacrifice of an animal, public prayer, and processions in which participants wore costumes and masks to ward off demons. On occasion athletic contests were part of the festivals.

Ludi consisted of circus games and theatrical plays. Of the circus games, chariot racing was, by far, the most popular. Held in the **Circus Maximus,** with an estimated seating ca-pacity of 150,000 to 250,00, the races were all-day affairs in which spectators, draped in red, white, blue, or green to identify with the faction (stable) of their favorite charioteer,

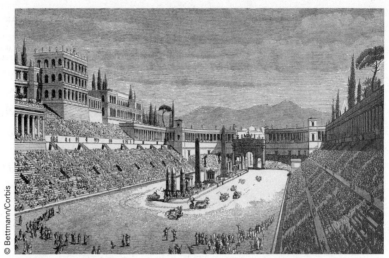

© Bettmann/Corbis

Of the circus games, Roman chariot racing was the most popular.

witnessed twenty-four races, each lasting about fifteen minutes in the seven-lap, five-mile race around the arena's spina, a thick, wall-like structure that separated both sides of the track. Between races, trick riders, boxers, and wrestlers entertained the huge audience. Stage plays began as flute dances, but later changed to mime, pantomime, comedies, and tragedies with regular plots. At times, an unfortunate criminal felt the pain of execution live on stage when a sinister plot called for a murder or homicide.

The *munera,* however, were the most extravagant spectacles, featuring **gladiatorial combat,** wild beast fights, and mock naval battles that thrilled spectators in the 50,000-seat **Colosseum.** Most gladiators came from the ranks of captured prisoners, criminals, or slaves. But freemen, too, in quest of fame and potential fortune, sometimes enrolled for training at gladiator schools. After undergoing assiduous training, gladiators were sold or rented to sponsors of games. They fought once or twice a year. Fights to the death were rare, particularly during the Empire, but blood-spilling injuries were common. In a symbolic carryover from Etruscan culture, the Romans viewed blood spilled during gladiatorial combat as nourishing the souls of the deceased in the next world. Meanwhile, successful gladiators attracted a public following that enabled them to generate lucrative earnings.

Gladiators dueled in pairs and sometimes in large groups. On occasion women, too, battled one another in the arena. Some female fighters were brought in from Ethiopia, but most were broad-shouldered Germanic women from the north. Sometimes gladiators slaughtered animals. Wild beast fights pitted animals against animals, soldiers against animals, and weaponless Christians against animals. Lions, leopards, and elephants were imported from Africa for these events. Tigers came from India, and wild boar from northern Europe. For mock naval battles, the Romans flooded the floor of the Colosseum and placed criminals on boats to slaughter each other, to the delight of the crowd. In some instances, Roman soldiers assaulted a mock town inhabited with criminals and slaves.

The existence of those spectacles is far less important than the reasons for their existence. The spectacles offered their sponsors the potential of political gain. Emperors gave games to remain popular with the people; in addition, they wanted to put themselves on display to show their followers they were in good health and still in control. With insurrection a constant fear, emperors believed they could keep the populace in check by occupying their time with games and satisfying their hunger with bread. The *panem et circensis* ("bread and circus") theme echoes true.

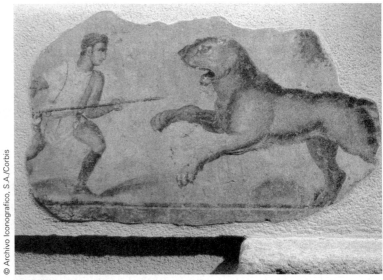

© Archivo Iconografico, S.A./Corbis

Roman gladiators.

The lowest-level politician, the *aedile* (or tribune) looked after the city, markets, and games. Tribunes sought higher political positions and sponsored games to secure enough support and votes to move into the higher echelons of consul (one of two chief magistrates who oversaw the state and army) or praetor (judicial officer). After serving in these positions, they then were appointed to governorships of newly conquered territories where they could reap immense riches. They would need this wealth, of course, to repay their creditors from whom they borrowed heavily in order to put on the games and spectacles as budding politicians. Emperors, too, strained Rome's treasury with their penchant for chariot races and gladiatorial combat or other extravaganzas in the Colosseum.[15]

On the Web

http://minbar.cs.dartmouth.edu/greecom/olympics/
Virtual museum of ancient Olympic games; discusses history, contests, victors, and competitors.

http://hickoksports.com/history/olancien.shtml
Contains historical sketches of ancient Olympic games.

http://olympics.Tufts.edu
Highly informative site. Perseus project with information about ancient Olympics, tour of Olympia, context of games, Olympic spirit, athletes' stories.

http://eawc.evansville.edu
Contains eight sites about the ancient world: Near East, India, Egypt, China, Greece, and Rome.

www.fhw.gr/projects/olympics
The Foundation of the Hellenic World has information on the ancient and modern games.

www.roman-empire.net/index.html
Excellent site for information about games and spectacles of Rome as well as the facilities where they took place—Colosseum, Circus Maximus, and the like.

www.upenn.edu/museum/Olympics
Contains information on daily life, work, religion, Olympics, and other aspects of life in Greece and Rome.

Key Terms

arête Greek conception of excellence in all facets of life: physical, intellectual, and spiritual. An ideal that Greeks strove for, but few ever reached it (page 29).

Campus Martius Parade ground where youth and men trained and developed their military skills (page 32).

Circus Maximus Largest arena in Rome, where chariot races were held before an estimated 150,000 to 250,000 spectators (page 32).

Colosseum Prominent arena in Rome where gladiatorial combat was held (page 33).

crown games Panhellenic athletic competitions held during non-Olympic years at Delphi, Corinth, and Nemea (page 28).

Festival of Sed Egyptian festival during which pharaohs ran on semicircular tracks to demonstrate their physical attributes and symbolically to renew their strength (page 22).

gladiatorial combat Fights, sometimes to the death, between two or more gladiators who were trained in the use of a variety of weapons (page 33).

gymnasia Public buildings in city-states where male Greek citizens participated in exercises, boxing, wrestling, pentathlon, and *pankration* (page 25).

Heraia Athletic competition (prenuptial rites of passage) for adolescent women held at Olympia one month before the Olympic Games (page 30).

mancalo Board game played by people of sub-Saharan Africa that involved placing objects in strategic positions to capture opponents' objects (page 23).

Olympic Games In ancient Greece, the primary festival consisting of athletic competitions held every forty-eight lunar months (page 26).

palestra Literally, a wrestling school; a place, generally private, where young Greek boys were taught the skills of wrestling by a trainer known as a *paidotribe* (page 25).

Panathenaic Festival One of the most prominent of ancient Greece's local festivals held at Athens (page 28).

pankration Athletic contest that involves elements of boxing, wrestling, and kicking. Victory requires the submission of one of the contestants (page 27).

pentathlon Athletic contest in which five events are performed: foot race, discus, javelin, long jump, and wrestling. The first contestant to win three events was declared the winner (page 26).

yoga In India and Asia, the practice of spiritual cleansing through meditation (page 22).

zane Statue erected at Olympia in the image of the god Zeus, to memorialize for posterity those who cheated at the Olympic Games (page 28).

Multiple Choice Questions

1. In ancient China the primary focus of physical activity was preparation for
   a. competitive sport
   b. leisure time pursuits
   c. betting and gambling
   d. military training
   e. all of the above

2. Meditation, deep breathing, and bodily contortions associated with yoga were commonly found in the ancient culture of
   a. Japan
   b. India
   c. Africa
   d. Mesopotamia
   e. Egypt

3. The connection between sport and ritual was readily seen in ancient Egypt when pharaohs participated in
   a. the Festival of Sed
   b. pyramid building
   c. the Feast of Ra
   d. stick fighting on the Nile
   e. camel races in Cairo

4. For sub-Saharan Africans, the activity that was an expressive art form with recreational, ceremonial, and ritualistic meanings was
   a. stick fighting
   b. fishing
   c. top spinning
   d. hunting
   e. dance

5. *Arête* means
   a. excellence
   b. happiness
   c. good and beautiful
   d. love
   e. none of the above

6. The ancient Greek city-state that gave women the most rights was

    a. Athens
    b. Sparta
    c. Corinth
    d. Epidauras
    e. Piraeus

7. The olive wreath given to victors at Olympic had little face value, but its symbolic value was great because victorious athletes often received

    a. free meals for life
    b. a *zane* for all time
    c. place of honor in their city-state
    d. a and c of the above
    e. a, b, and c of the above

8. When athletes realized that winning brought them bountiful rewards, they traveled around Greece entering as many different competitions as they could and came to be known as

    a. model athletes
    b. divine athletes
    c. tramp athletes
    d. secular athletes
    e. none of the above

9. The lowest political office-holders in Rome who aspired to the higher positions were

    a. consuls
    b. *praetors*
    c. governors
    d. *aediles*
    e. emperors

10. The political office-holders in question 9 believed they could increase their popularity and thus move into the higher positions by

    a. mugging emperors
    b. pushing drugs
    c. turning letters
    d. sponsoring games
    e. driving chariots

Critical Thinking Questions

1. Sporting activities and athletic competition are prominent components of human nature because they seem to satisfy our "competitive instincts." Why were they present in all the cultures covered in this chapter, and what purposes did they serve?

2. In most ancient Greek city-states and in ancient Rome, women found themselves in subservient childbearing, child-rearing roles. Why do you suppose women were relegated to this position in ancient cultures and—given the political, social, and economic structure of the ancient world—indicate how women might have been able to remove themselves from this position.

3. Olympic contestants who were caught cheating at Olympia were memorialized for posterity when their names were carved on pedestal supporting a statue of Zeus, called a *zane*. Why were there only eleven *zanes* in nearly 1,200 years of Olympic competition?

4. The ancient Olympic Games began in 776 B.C.E. and continued until 394 C.E. What forces brought about the downfall of the ancient Olympics and Greek athletics in general, and why couldn't the Olympic movement initiated by the ancient Greeks survive beyond the ancient period?

5. Romans enjoyed watching chariot racing, gladiatorial combat, wild beast fights, and other spectacles better than actually participating in athletic contests. What was it about Roman life and culture that led them to such passive entertainment and why were so many spectacles held in ancient Rome?

Notes and References

1. Michael Speak, "Recreation and Sport in Ancient China," in *Sport and Physical Education in China*, edited by James Riordan and Robin Jones (London: Spon Press, 1999), 26–37.

2. Deobold D. Van Dalen and Bruce L. Bennett, *A World History of Physical Education*, 2d ed. (Englewood Cliffs, N.J.: Prentice-Hall, Inc, 1971), 19–24.

3. Robert A. Mechikoff and Steven Estes, *A History and Philosophy of Sport and Physical Education*, 3rd ed. (Boston: WCB McGraw-Hill, 2002), 25–27.

4. Wolfgang Decker, *Sport and Games of Ancient Egypt,* translated by Allen Guttmann (New Haven: Yale University Press, 1992), 24–38, 71–89, 158–66.

5. James Blacking, "Games and Sport in Pre-Colonial African Societies"; Sigfried Paul, "The Wrestling Tradition and Its Social Functions"; Thomas Q. Reefe, "The Biggest Game of All: Gambling in Traditional Africa" in *Sport in Africa: Essays in Social History,* edited by William J. Baker and James Mangan (New York: Africana, 1987), 3–18, 23–42, 47–70.

6. Mark Golden, *Sport and Society in Ancient Greece* (Cambridge: Cambridge University Press, 1998), 88–93.

7. Michael Poliakoff, *Combat Sports of the Ancient World* (New Haven: Yale University Press, 1987), 89–108, 117–33.

8. David C. Young, *The Olympic Myth of Greek Amateur Athletics* (Chicago: Ares, 1989), 128–33.

9. Ibid., 134–46.

10. Allen Guttmann, *Women's Sports, A History* (New York: Columbia University Press, 1991), 22.

11. Ibid., 17-32.

12. Lionel Casson, *Everyday Life in Ancient Rome,* rev. ed. (Baltimore: Johns Hopkins University Press, 1975), 1–9; Chester G. Stark, *The Ancient Romans* (New York: Oxford University Press, 1971), 9–23.

13. J. F. Dobson, *Ancient Education and Its Meaning to Us* (New York: Cooper Square, 1963); Lionel Casson, *Everyday Life in Ancient Rome,* rev. ed. (Baltimore: Johns Hopkins University Press, 1975), 1–9; Chester G. Stark, *The Ancient Romans* (New York: Oxford University Press, 1971), 9–23, 105–17; Guttmann, 34.

14. Guttmann, 38.

15. J. P. V. D. Balsdon, *Life and Leisure in Ancient Rome* (New York: McGraw-Hill, 1969), 244–53, 268, 270–77, 291, 308–12; Guttmann, 39.

3

SPORTS, GAMES, AND IDEOLOGY: THE MIDDLE AGES TO THE AGE OF EUROPEAN NATIONALISM

Chapter Objectives

After reading this chapter, the student will be able to

- Discuss at least two ways in which physical activity was used during the Middle Ages

- Describe the concept of the human body during the Middle Ages

- Define humanism and its meaning in Renaissance thought

- Describe the contributions of Jean-Jacques Rousseau to physical education

- Define nationalism and explain its relationship to Friedrich Jahn's turnverein

- Discuss the evolution of German gymnastics

- Describe the evolution and direction of Swedish gymnastics

MEDIEVAL LIFE AND THE SYSTEM OF FEUDALISM

With the fall of the Roman Empire at the end of the fifth century, Western civilization experienced a period of turmoil and had to reconstitute itself. Chaos reigned as hordes of barbarians—Goths, Huns, Vandals, Lombards, Saxons and others—ravaged the remains of Rome. In Roman army towns and outposts, local inhabitants replaced Roman customs and Latin with their own practices and native language. The strongest, most powerful individuals attracted followers and occupied territory that they could control, which eventually became their fiefs or manors. In time the lord of the manor erected a fortress (ultimately, a castle) for protection against invaders. In exchange for the lord's protection, serfs tilled the soil and carried out other domestic duties necessary to sustain life on the manor. As the lord increased his power and stature, he expanded his domain by conquering the territory of neighboring lords. He then appointed his most trusted knights (vassals) to oversee newly captured lands. For each territorial acquisition, the lord selected another vassal to oversee the new possession. This system of **feudalism** prevailed for nearly a thousand years and ultimately led to the development of nation-states in the fourteenth and fifteenth centuries.

THE PREVALENCE AND IMPACT OF CHRISTIANITY

After gaining a stronghold in Rome, Christianity swept through medieval Europe. For the medieval peasant whose life was filled with toil and strife, and little hope for improvement, the expectation of eternity offered reason to endure the daily grind. People embraced Christianity because salvation of the soul was the highest priority. Monasteries and castles dotted the medieval landscape. Religious orders emerged; monks and nuns shunned the secular world and often turned to **asceticism,** with vows of obedience, poverty, and celibacy. Catholicism emphasized spiritual development and suppression of animal instincts.

The conversion of temporal leaders, like Charlemagne, to Christianity insured the Church's hold on the European continent. This mutually beneficial relationship between temporal lord and religious cleric solidified the control each had over the populace. In many regions, the dominant lords eventually became kings or emperors, who, with their legions of knights, defended the faith and protected their subjects.

CHIVALRY AND THE LURE OF KNIGHTHOOD

Preparation and training for knighthood was a difficult task that involved considerable sacrifice. Generally, each vassal's eldest son was sent to the lord's castle for training. There he learned military skills essential for warfare and court manners, but he also had to endure elements of asceticism— lengthy periods of fasting, solitude, and prayer vigils—before gaining admission into the sanctum of knighthood. Ideally, the knight was supposed to be well-rounded—a paragon of physical prowess and stamina; a font of intelligence blended with courage, virtue, and good manners; and a beacon of enthusiasm eager to defend Christianity. Despite the way knights are romanticized in folklore and literature, very few ever achieved the ideal. In fact, a large number, particularly the Crusaders, assaulted and raped innocent victims and pillaged peaceful villages in the name of Christianity.

To maintain the proficiency of their military and fighting skills, knights participated in **tournaments** and **melees.** In

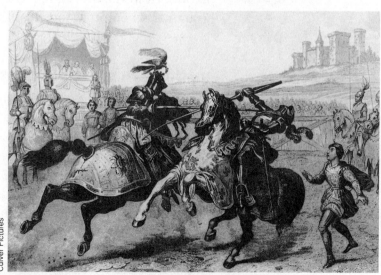

Medieval knights participated in tournaments and melees.

a **joust,** two knights with lances tried to unseat each other from their horses, while in a melee two teams of knights simultaneously jousted against each other. Jousting continued into the fifteenth century, when armor-piercing weapons and new battlefield strategies made it obsolete.[1]

EDUCATION DURING THE MIDDLE AGES

Even more than knighthood, Christianity played an important role in medieval education. During the early Middle Ages (or the Dark Ages as the fifth to ninth centuries are sometimes called), the monasteries established schools to educate monks and youth preparing to be monks. The chief purpose of **monastic schools** was to teach monks and novitiates to read scripture. Some schools even accepted lay students from privileged families. Students were schooled in the Seven Liberal Arts: the *trivium* (grammar, rhetoric, and logic) and the *quadrivium* (arithmetic, geometry, astronomy, and music). Later, when cathedrals sprung up in cities across Europe, schools were established there, too, to train clerics for each bishopric (or diocese). These schools also attracted lay students. Neither the monastic nor the **cathedral schools** had any provisions for physical education, nor were they concerned about the physical attributes of human nature. However, they did lay the groundwork for the early grammar schools that served as the foundation of our modern system of education.[2]

RISE OF CITIES AND UNIVERSITIES

Most cities emerged as marketplaces at strategic sites along a river, at a crossroads, or at an accessible seacoast harbor. As east-west trade expanded, due in part to the Crusades, so did cities. Some became seats of a manor; others became ecclesiastical centers; still others became nexuses of trade. In fostering commerce, merchants planted the seeds of capitalism and came to dominate the economy of emerging cities and towns. They extracted benefits from the nobility that gave them more rights and freedom. Craftspersons (carpenters, masons, glaziers, blacksmiths, and so on) and peasants who could leave the manor (some serfs were granted freedom;

others escaped and gained their independence if they could remain undetected for a year and a day) migrated to cities where they could apply and market their skills in exchange for a better lifestyle and the greater freedom that cities offered. Craftspeople banded together and formed guilds that enhanced their opportunities and benefits.

Scholars, too, organized themselves into guilds, and from those guilds came the university. The earliest universities had no buildings. Initially, a master lecturer either rented a room or made space in his home for lecturing. Eventually, several master lecturers pooled their resources and rented a storefront or part of a building. Gradually, as more lecturers joined forces, an entire building was acquired for education. Growing enrollments and increased revenue enabled universities to secure additional buildings, giving each institution its own identity within a city. Some universities grew out of cathedral schools. The principal subjects were the arts, theology, law, and medicine.[3]

There were no provisions for physical education. Consequently, students often grew rowdy as stored-up energy accumulated from successive hours of lectures. Misdeeds often led to pranks and fights among students. On occasion aggressive behavior escalated into brawls with townspeople. The St. Scholastica's Day riot in 1354 went from a quarrel to an armed battle that left many wounded and several dead. Not all incidents stemming from unexpended energy had negative results. In some instances students played football (soccer) games that soon developed into natural rivalries in which students from the same geographical regions challenged students from another region.[4]

HOLIDAYS AND FESTIVALS

The difficulty of life in the Middle Ages was reflected in the number of holy days and feast days on the medieval calendar. Holy days (which would later become holidays) and feast days were excuses to celebrate and helped the people to cope with drudgery. Originally scheduled around agrarian seasonal cycles, holy days and festivals revolved around planting, harvesting, Christmas, and pre-Lenten festivities.

Celebrations began with church services, prayer, and spiritual hymns and soon turned to entertainment with jugglers, minstrels, and troubadours. Gambling was prevalent; dancing was popular; prostitution available; and animal baits, cock fighting, and football were common practices. At times university students joined in the fun and celebrated with townspeople. Football games often pitted men of one parish against those of another or the marrieds against the bachelors. The games were more of a free-for-all than contests of skill, yet they served as a means of escaping the rigors of life.[5]

RENAISSANCE THOUGHT AND HUMANISTIC LEANINGS

As trade exposed Western society to other cultures, knowledge and the quest for information increased. There was an infatuation with and renewed interest in Greek and Roman classics. Scholars of the **Renaissance** period read and translated Greek works that portrayed the human body as an instrument of beauty. Renaissance scholars and artists respected and admired the human form, even though they still viewed the soul still as holding the passport to salvation. In Renaissance painting and sculpture, full-length images of the human body appeared vibrant and robust in comparison with the medieval images inspired by spiritual themes; these often represented only a person's head or showed angelic figures with wings.

HUMANIST LEADERS

Renaissance thought produced humanists whose interest in the body triggered a revival of Greek gymnastics, an effective mechanism in the ancient world for developing and maintaining physical attributes. The thrust toward **humanism** was confirmed in the actions of Vittorino da Feltre (1378–1446), Aeneas Sylvius Piccolomini (Pope Pius II; 1405–1464), and Hieronymus Mercurialis (1530–1606). Da Feltre opened a court school, La Giocosa, at Mantua. It contained spacious, well-ventilated rooms for indoor programs and meadows and woods for outdoor activities. He promoted exercise during all seasons and stressed natural activities of running, jumping, and hiking, along with ball games, fencing, and riding. He taught a manual of arms to those destined for military service and gymnastics to those who would follow a civilian lifestyle. He advocated individualized instruction and hired a large staff to keep class enrollments low so teachers could get to know students personally. Da Feltre's program enabled teachers to plan exercise programs in accordance with the needs of the students. Its versatility accommodated those with special needs, particularly the physically challenged.

Self-activity and self-expression were important to humanists. Pius II, in a marked departure from his papal predecessors, encouraged racing, dancing, and swimming for men and women. He believed that games and exercise would strengthen youth, improve posture, and promote dignity. Mercurialis, an Italian physician, wrote favorably about Greek gymnastics in his *De Arte Gymnastica* and stressed the value of exercise for hygienic purposes.[6]

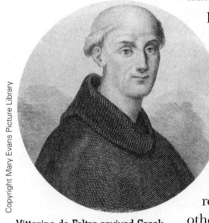

Copyright Mary Evans Picture Library

Vittorino da Feltre revived Greek gymnastics at his La Giocosa court school.

In northern Europe, humanists followed the lead of Desiderius Erasmus (c. 1466–1536), who championed reform through education. While he was not directly an ally of physical activity, his writings attracted others with interests in physical exercise to the humanistic movement. Two of his most notable disciples were Sir Thomas Elyot and Roger Ascham. Elyot, while serving in the court of Henry VIII, developed an interest in the education of courtiers. He recommended running, hunting, hawking, wrestling (with proper precautions), lifting and throwing heavy stones, using dumbbells, playing tennis, swimming, and dancing. For military purposes he proclaimed the benefits of riding, fencing, and mastering the battle-axe and longbow. Ascham, a tutor of Elizabeth I, promoted running, jumping, leaping, wrestling, swimming, dancing, tennis, hunting, and hawking as recreational pursuits in his book, *The Schoolmaster.* For military preparedness he called for proficiency at the tilting ring and in archery and weaponry. Both men believed these skills were necessary for courtly manners as well as military protection.

Another early humanist, Baldassare Castiglione, in his *Book of the Courtier* (1528), envisioned the ideal courtier as strong, flexible, quick, and elusive. In addition, the courtier needed great stamina and knowledge of wrestling, jousting, tilting, fencing, and horse riding. He also practiced running and leaping for agility and stamina, swimming for survival training, and dance for grace and manners.[7]

REFORMATION AND REALISM

Concern for weaponry and the call for arms was evident in John Milton's *Tractate on Education,* in which he advises a friend to educate his son by teaching him weapons' skills, riding, and wrestling. At the time, England was experiencing a period of religious turmoil, and Milton, with his Puritan leanings, advocated preparation in martial skills, so Puritan youth would be able to fend off the forces of the Crown.

On the European continent, Martin Luther raised other kinds of issues in questioning papal authority and identifying the abuses of Catholic clergy—the first steps toward the Protestant **Reformation.** In Luther's mind, the pleasure and enjoyment derived from physical activity could serve as a palliative for eschewing evil temptations. To that extent, he recommended fencing, wrestling, and gymnastics. Moreover, strong, healthy bodies and untarnished minds enabled one to perform daily labor more effectively and to serve the Lord more fully. And from a humanistic viewpoint, the strong and healthy also possess the energy and drive to help the infirm and those less fortunate.[8]

François Rabelais (1483–1553), Richard Mulcaster (1530–1611), and Michel de Montaigne (1553–1592) believed in preparing individuals for the challenges of the secular world through education. They thought that social, moral, spiritual, and physical components of education were essential to the total development of the individual. Horse riding, fencing, hunting, ball playing, running, and swimming were among the activities promoted for physical development. Experience is critical for the learning process and just as important as book learning for carrying out life tasks. Although Rabelais's ideas for school reform fell upon deaf ears during his lifetime, he had a significant influence upon Montaigne, Locke, and Rousseau. Among Mulcaster's many traits was his concern for equality in education. He wanted females to have the same opportunities as males and the poor to receive the same schooling as the wealthy. He wanted education to focus on the child rather than the subject. Montaigne believed in vigorous exercise and strict discipline for developing manly characteristics. Resurrecting Sparta's stern training methods, Montaigne's program called for exposing youth to the elements of cold, heat, wind, rain, and sun. Austerity training would strengthen character and protect the soul. John Locke (1632–1704), borrowing a page from Montaigne, promoted exposure to environmental elements as well. In *Some Thoughts on Education,* he also raised issues of health and nutrition and asserted that the body had to be strong in order for the mind to develop. Physical activity stimulates the body and refreshes the mind. For Montaigne, it was also a foundation upon which moral and intellectual training could be built.[9]

AGE OF ENLIGHTENMENT

Growing out of Renaissance thought and criticism of the absolute power of both church and state was the **Enlightenment,** whose thought embodied (1) the inalienable rights of humankind and (2) humanity's mastery of its own environment through critical analysis and scientific investigation. In his classics, *Discourse on Inequality* and *The Social Contract,* Jean-Jacques Rousseau (1712–1788) elevated the dignity of humankind and affected the course of Western history. His work in the educational sphere, *Emile,* had significant implications for the inclusion of physical activity in the educative process. A proponent of naturalism, Rousseau espoused natural activities of running, jumping, climbing, and throwing—outdoors, where the senses of sight, sound, and touch could be part of the learning experience. The interaction with nature in an outdoor environment facilitated the learning process. Reinforcing his naturalistic leanings, Rousseau offered an analogy in which he compared peasants with

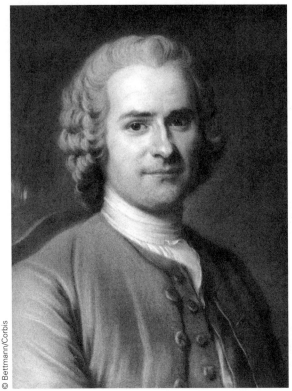

Jean-Jacques Rousseau spearheaded the movement toward sense learning and natural activities.

savages in an educational forum. Peasants are creatures of routine who accept whatever is presented without thinking, whereas savages must invoke their creative and imaginative powers in order to survive. Their ingenuity and creative ability to solve problems enable them to adapt to the vicissitudes of life. Clearly, Rousseau wanted Emile and students of all dimensions to assume the posture of his figurative savage. Rousseau was a font of ideas for others to consider and implement.[10]

Johann Basedow (1723–1790) was the first educator to apply Rousseau's ideas in an educational setting when he opened his school, the Philanthropinum, in 1774 at Dessau. He stressed learning through the senses in natural settings. His students wore simple uniforms, rather than the stiff, formal regalia in vogue at the time, for freedom of movement as prescribed in *Emile*. The ten-hour day at Basedow's institution consisted of five hours of intellectual studies, two hours of manual labor (carpentry, masonry, and the like), and three hours of physical activities. Young students engaged in running, wrestling, throwing, and jumping, while the older students participated in fencing, riding, vaulting, dancing, and music. Johann Simon, instructor at the Philanthropinum, was the mastermind behind the curriculum, which arranged age-appropriate activities based on the students' needs and maturation level. Insufficient financial resources forced the school to close in 1793.[11]

A second German school modeled after Basedow's Philanthropinum was the Schnepfenthal Educational Institute founded by Christian Salzmann. Johann Guts Muths (1759–1839) taught physical education there for more than fifty years and is credited with laying the foundation for German gymnastics. He constructed outdoor apparatus for climbing, swinging, and vaulting. His program incorporated natural activities of all types—walking, running, jumping, thrusting, pulling, pushing, balancing, lifting, carrying, throwing, wrestling, dancing, and swimming. The school emphasized personal health; diet was simple, but nutritious. The Institute was well-ventilated and well-lighted. Guts Muths believed in strengthening the body first, so it could accommodate the maturing mind. He also advocated physical activities for girls and women.[12]

More than any other educator, Johann Heinrich Pestalozzi (1746–1827) carried Rousseau's ideas to fruition at his school at Yverdon, where he combined intellectual, moral, and practical components of education. The latter involved manual labor and physical education. Vocational training and physical education, along with intellectual studies and morality training, enabled students to develop to their fullest potential. Fostering the conception of "unity of the child," Pestalozzi channeled his students toward gymnastics, hiking, swimming, sledding, skating, dancing, and fencing. "Object teaching," through the use of picture

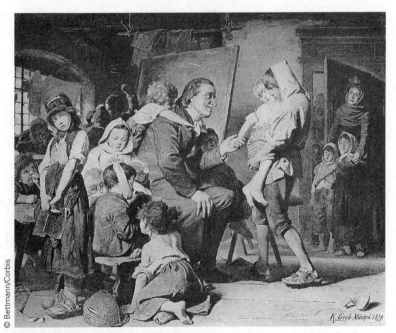

Johann Heinrich Pestalozzi put Rousseau's ideas into practice at this school in Yverdon.

books, heightened sensory learning. Military drill was part of the curriculum; and programs for women and girls were provided primarily for health and domestic purposes.

A contemporary of Pestalozzi's, Friedrich Froebel (1782–1852) saw redeeming social values in play. In fact, he viewed play as the highest form of child development. In his work, *The Education of Man,* Froebel proclaimed that self-activity through observation, discovery, and creativity contributes to the oneness of a person. Like Guts Muths and Pestalozzi, he believed that physical education could enhance intellectual faculties. He encouraged teachers and students to work together in a learning environment to enable the child to become a productive adult. His approach to play and physical activity as precepts to intellectual development was embodied in the kindergarten he created.[13]

GERMAN NATIONALISM

Friedrich Ludwig Jahn (1778–1852), a leader of German **nationalism,** believed that the German-speaking states should be united under the leadership of Prussia. When Prussia refused to join sixteen German sister states in support of Napoleon in 1804, the French general entered Prussia and defeated its army at the Battle of Jena, costing Prussia territories and the embarrassment of French occupation. Within Prussia, a resistance movement led to wars of liberation, from 1813 to 1815. Jahn was one of the principal agitators behind the resistance. After moving to Berlin in 1809, Jahn began teaching gymnastics and physical exercise and soon became associated with other German patriots. As a teacher of gymnastics, he erected outdoor apparatus, based on Guts Muths's model, and began to attract students to his program. In 1811 he organized the **turnverein** (gymnastics clubs) and instilled nationalistic pride into his students. He inspired the turners (members of the club) to join in the wars of liberation against French occupation. Following Napoleon's defeat and exile for a second time in 1815, Kaiser Friedrich Wilhelm III banned the turners on the advice of Austrian Prince Metternich because the gymnastics clubs were considered hotbeds of revolution.

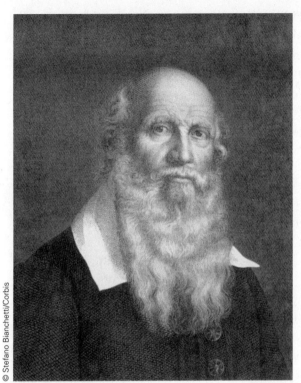

© Stefano Bianchetti/Corbis

Friedrich Ludwig Jahn, the German nationalist who founded the turnverein.

Jahn was imprisoned, then released, but he was placed under surveillance and banned from living in cities that housed universities or gymnasiums where he might foment revolution. Even though his turners were suppressed and Jahn was virtually sequestered for most of his adult life, the turner movement he initiated was the progenitor of a highly conditioned Prussian army that would dominate Europe in succeeding generations.[14]

SWEDISH AND DANISH GYMNASTICS

Nationalism and patriotism also extended to Sweden and Denmark during the turmoil created by the Napoleonic wars. As a consequence of supporting the defeated side, Denmark lost Norway to Sweden and other territory to England. Under the leadership of Franz Nachtegall (1777–1847), German gymnastics made their way into Denmark. After reading Guts Muths's *Gymnastics for Youth*, Nachtegall began teaching gymnastics along with other subjects to his tutorial pupils. In 1799 he opened a private gymnasium in Copenhagen that proved to be quite popular, and his methods spread to private and public school settings where he taught gymnastics. He used rope and hanging ladders, climbing poles, balance beam, and vaulting horses. As his program grew in popularity, he moved into a university environment where he became the director of the Military Gymnastic Institute. He was instrumental in establishing compulsory physical education laws for Danish schoolchildren. Instructors at the Military Gymnastic Institute were then trained to prepare teachers in military gymnastics, which ultimately replaced Guts Muths's system in Denmark.[15]

Swedish nationalist Per Henrik Ling (1776–1839) learned gymnastics from Nachtegall as a student at the university in Copenhagen. Ling also took up fencing, which fortuitously gave him relief from the arthritis that inflamed his arm. His curiosity led him to examine the medical effects of exercise, which eventually became the basis of his gymnastic system. Upon his return from Denmark, Ling introduced gymnastics to Sweden. Initially, though, Ling's gymnastics, supported and encouraged by King Charles XIV, took on a military orientation because Sweden had lost Finland to the Russians in 1808 and possessions south of the Baltic to Napoleon a year earlier. Ling's outlook on gymnastics was holistic: He advocated harmonious development of the body. He thus incorporated developmental, medical (corrective), military, and aesthetic components into his system. When the danger of foreign threats subsided, Ling's system evolved into educational and medical gymnastics. Less complicated than Jahn's German gymnastics, Ling's movements were more free exercises without hand-held apparatus. Among the apparatus he did employ were stall bars, window ladder, Swedish box, and oblique rope. One drawback was the uncomfortable, stretched-out positions that participants had to maintain while the instructor made corrections. Though not highly popular in Sweden, Ling's system spread to the United States, where it received a high degree of recognition during the late nineteenth century.[16]

On the Web

http://www.chronique.com
Offers information on knighthood, jousting, tournaments, and other facets of medieval life.

http://eawc.evansville.edu
Site on medieval Europe.

http://georgetown.edu/labyrinth
Site contains information about knighthood, chivalry, and tournaments.

http://learner.org/exhibits/renaissance
This site, developed by the Annenberg Foundation and the Corporation for Public Broadcasting, offers a guided tour of the Renaissance.

http://www.metmuseum.org/collections
The Metropolitan Museum of Art's site contains information on life, armor, and weapons during the Middle Ages.

http://www.netcrafters.net/jousting/history/medieval.htm
Contains information on the history of jousting and tournaments.

http://www.nga.gov
Site of the National Gallery of Art in Washington, D.C., that provides a
tour of the Renaissance through art.

www.womeninworldhistory.com/heroine3.htm
Site of Women in the World history curriculum. This article discusses
"women left behind" to defend castles and property during the Crusades.

Key Terms

asceticism Strong emphasis on humans' spiritual development and the
suppression of their animal instincts (page 42).

cathedral schools Established at cathedrals in medieval cities to train
clerics for each bishopric or diocese; they accepted lay students (page 44).

Enlightenment Eighteenth-century movement growing out of Renaissance;
it emphasized inalienable rights of humankind and its quest to master the
environment through critical analysis and scientific investigation (page 49).

feudalism A system of political organization in which the lord or king
held all land in fee; vassals (subordinates) administered and paid
homage to the lord with foods, clothing, and other goods; in return,
vassals and their tenants (serfs) received protection through the lord's
military legion (page 42).

humanism Intellectual and artistic movement that manifests a strong
interest in human nature, welfare of humanity, and appreciation for joy
and beauty in life (page 46).

joust Contest in which two knights tried to unseat each other from their
horses (page 44).

melee Contests in which teams of knights jousted simultaneously against
each other (page 43).

monastic schools Established in the monasteries to teach monks and
novitiates to read scripture; they sometimes accepted lay students from
privileged families (page 44).

nationalism Loyalty and devotion to one's country; pride in one's
homeland (page 52).

Reformation Religious movement in which the doctrine and practices of
the Roman Catholic Church were questioned; led to establishment of
Protestant denominations (page 48).

Renaissance Period in history between Middle Ages and modern period
(fourteenth to seventeenth centuries) characterized by the rebirth of
Greek and Roman art, literature, and ideology (page 46).

tournament Events in which knights maintained their military and fighting skills through jousting and melee contests (page 43).

turnverein Gymnastic clubs for German youth established by Friedrich Jahn in early nineteenth century as a reaction to Napoleon's conquests and occupation of Prussia (page 42).

Multiple Choice Questions

1. The medieval system of mutual protection based upon vassalage was
   a. feudalism
   b. humanism
   c. romanticism
   d. asceticism
   e. realism

2. Early medieval education was held in
   a. monastic schools
   b. gladiatorial schools
   c. public schools
   d. a and b of the above
   e. a, b, and c of the above

3. Emphasis on the spirit (soul) and the suppression of the physical and bodily needs is referred to as
   a. feudalism
   b. humanism
   c. romanticism
   d. asceticism
   e. realism

4. The French theorist who advocated physical development through the application of natural activities in the education of his model student, Emile, was:
   a. Michel de Montaigne
   b. François Rabelais
   c. Baldassare Castiglione
   d. Jean-Jacques Rousseau
   e. Rene Descartes

5. The first educator to apply Rousseau's ideas in an educational setting at his school, the Philanthropinum, was
   a. Johann Basedow
   b. Heinrich Pestalozzi
   c. Friedrich Jahn
   d. Johann Guts Muths
   e. Friedrich Froebel

6. The instructor at the Schnepfenthal who constructed outdoor climbing and vaulting apparatus and is credited with laying the foundation for German gymnastics was

    a. Johann Basedow
    b. Heinrich Pestalozzi
    c. Friedrich Jahn
    d. Johann Guts Muths
    e. Friedrich Froebel

7. The educator who applied Rousseau's ideas to their fullest extent when he combined intellectual, moral and practical components of education at this school in Yverdon was

    a. Johann Basedow
    b. Heinrich Pestalozzi
    c. Friedrich Jahn
    d. Johann Guts Muths
    e. Friedrich Froebel

8. The gymnastics clubs organized by the German nationalist, Friedrich Jahn, were called

    a. kindergarten
    b. volkesport
    c. korperscultur
    d. biergarten
    e. turnverein

9. The individual who promoted gymnastics in Sweden initially for military purposes and later for educational and rehabilitative reasons was

    a. Per Henrik Ling
    b. Friedrich Jahn
    c. Friedrich Wilhelm IV
    d. Adolf Spiess
    e. Metternich

10. The individual who introduced German gymnastics in Denmark and later with modifications developed the Danish system was

    a. Per Henrik Ling
    b. Friedrich Jahn
    c. Friedrich Wilhelm IV
    d. Johann Guts Muths
    e. Franz Nachtegall

Critical Thinking Questions

1. Knights and knighthood have been depicted in Western literature as well-mannered, gentlemanly figures who exhibited courage, protected women, and defended the Church (think of King Arthur, Sir Lancelot, Sir Gawain, and Ivanhoe). From your knowledge of human nature,

along with this chapter's analysis of medieval life, provide a realistic view of the medieval knight and explain why few, if any knights, ever reached the ideal pinnacle we often read about in the literature.

2. Why did medieval university students often turn to rowdyism and violent behavior, and what measures could college administrators have taken to defuse the students' aberrant behavior?

3. Discuss how the revival of Greek and Roman thought, literature, and education during the Renaissance influenced humankind's view of the human body and the direction of education during that time period.

4. Jean-Jacques Rousseau compared students to peasants, creatures of routine, and to savages, who had to rely on their own resourcefulness to survive. What kind of student did Rousseau want? Explain why, and then indicate how today's students might reflect Rousseau's analogy.

5. The political-military climate of nineteenth-century Europe led to the evolution and development of German and Swedish gymnastics. Why did Swedish gymnastics adopt educational and medical components when German gymnastics continued with a militaristic orientation?

Notes and References

1. William J. Baker, *Sports in the Modern World*, rev. ed. (Urbana: University of Illinois Press, 1988), 49–53.

2. Deobold D. Van Dalen and Bruce L. Bennett, *A World History of Physical Education*, 2d ed. (Englewood Cliffs, N.J.: Prentice-Hall, 1971), 19–24.

3. Hastings Rashdall, *The Universities of Europe during the Middle Ages* (Oxford: Clarendon Press, 1936).

4. Ibid., 120–21.

5. Baker, 43–49.

6. Ellen W. Gerber, *Innovators and Institutions in Physical Education* (Philadelphia: Lea & Febiger, 1971), 22–50.

7. Robert A. Mechikoff and Steven Estes, *A History and Philosophy of Sport and Physical Education*, 3rd ed. (Boston: WCB McGraw-Hill, 2002), 111–19.

8. Van Dalen and Bennett, 144–46.

9. Gerber, 54–75.

10. Rousseau, Jean-Jacques, *Emile*, 52–55.

11. Mechikoff and Estes, 139–140.

12. Van Dalen and Bennett, 189–92.

13. Gerber, 87–99

14. Van Dalen and Bennett, 204–14.

15. Ibid., 255–59.

16. Ibid., 236–40.

4

AMERICAN PHYSICAL EDUCATION AND PHYSICAL ACTIVITY BEFORE 1900

Chapter Objectives

After reading this chapter, the student will be able to

- Identify at least four European contributions to American physical education

- List at least one contribution of Catharine Beecher, Elizabeth Blackwell, Sylvester Graham, William Alcott, and Dioclesian Lewis

- Differentiate between German and Swedish gymnastics in terms of purpose and style

- List at least one contribution of Edward Hitchcock, Dudley Sargent, Amy Morris Homans, Delphine Hanna, and William G. Anderson

- Explain the process by which AAHPERD and the profession of physical education was founded

- Identify at least three forces that led to the emergence of intercollegiate athletics

GAMES AND ACTIVITIES OF NATIVE AMERICANS

Long before Europeans discovered the Americas, Indian tribes inhabited the lands of the Western hemisphere. As with other cultures, physical activity served several purposes for American Indians. **Lacrosse, shinny** (or bandy, as this Indian version of field hockey was called), and other games of dexterity enabled Native Americans to sharpen their survival skills, to conduct ceremonies embedded in their ritual, and to seek and satisfy their quest for excitement. On horseback and on foot, Indians honed their self-protective and hunting skills with target games involving arrows, spears, and other objects. Ceremonies offered to supernatural powers in order to insure a bountiful hunt, sufficient rainfall, or wartime success often combined vigorous games with elements of dance ritual. In Mexico and Central America, Aztec and Mayan Indians played a rigorous ball game on a court shaped like a block letter I. Rules of **court ball** are sketchy at best, but some versions called for the players to propel a rubber ball (about the size of a softball) through a ring without using their hands or feet. With just one ball for a cadre of players, the game took on

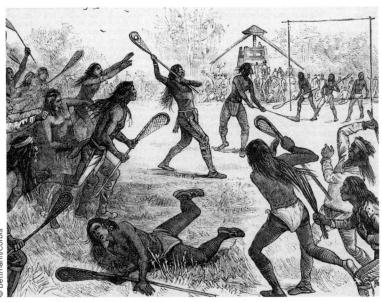

© Bettmann/Corbis

American Indians playing lacrosse.

an atmosphere of a close combat free-for-all that no doubt refined their battle skills.

Indians throughout the Western hemisphere played games of calculation and chance in addition to those vigorous games demanding physical prowess. Two popular gambling games were bowls, a form of dice with knuckle bones, and staves, a set of sticks with decorative and plain sides. Players rolled the staves onto the ground from an animal skin and scored points when all of one side or equal numbers of both sides turned up. Indians were occupied in games such as these when new faces from the European continent appeared on their shores.

COLONIAL LIFESTYLES AND SPORTING PRACTICES

The discovery of the New World brought explorers from Spain, France, Holland, and England. While the Spaniards searched for gold and the French hunted for fur, the English colonized the land that would eventually become the United States and, in doing so, left their imprint on American culture and life in the form of language, customs, common law, style of government, and educational system. It is not surprising, then, that approximately two-thirds of our sports and recreational activities come from England.

The English settled initially in 1607 at Jamestown in Virginia, then in 1620 in Massachusetts, and later in other areas. In both early colonies, life was a struggle until the colonists could sustain themselves. All energy had to go into the survival effort, with no time for sport or recreation. In fact, the Jamestown settlers banned sports and games for that reason, but once the colony established itself on firm footing, the ban was lifted and sports and games became commonplace. The Southern lifestyle, with its plantation economy, contributed to the establishment of slavery, which was introduced to the New World in 1619, a year before the Pilgrims landed at Plymouth. Slavery, in turn, gave rise to a planter aristocracy with ample leisure for partaking in sports and recreational activities.

On the other hand, the Massachusetts colonists, steeped in Calvinism, opposed most sports because they conflicted with their narrow social ethic of industry, piety, and frugality. Popularly known as the Puritan ethic, this combination of hard work, prayer, and righteousness, as well as financial prudence, sought to create a productive society. Because sport, for the most part, was unproductive (it had no end product), Puritans equated it with idleness, or the work of the devil. Hence its prohibition, except for what they considered to be "rational recreations," swimming, running, ice skating, and the like, which had self-improvement benefits.

As Massachusetts Bay's population swelled by 16,000 during the 1630s due to the "Great Migration," Puritans found themselves in a minority, but they maintained control of the colony by holding important governmental positions. They also controlled the colony's most important social institution, the Congregational Church, which they kept exclusive. Realizing that the majority needed social outlets, they permitted, and some of them even owned, taverns. Out of the tavern atmosphere sprouted a host of sporting and recreational activities, including turkey shoots, cock fighting, animal baiting, and horse racing. Colony officials and magistrates often turned their backs on these activities, rather than create unrest among the majority of residents.[1]

The tavern played a less visible role in the development of sport in the South. In a region dominated by a planter aristocracy, the Southern gentry pursued such exclusive sporting activities as fox hunting and **ring tourneys.** The latter was a modern rendition of medieval jousting in which a rider at full gallop attempted to insert a lance into a tiny suspended ring. Then, too, the gambling element of horse racing and cock fighting aroused the betting juices of Southern gentlemen who patronized these sporting activities in which slaves, freed blacks, and poor whites often trained the animals.

In addition to sporting activities, the English brought their education system to America. Massachusetts Bay took the lead in establishing elementary and Latin grammar schools in its communities. This trend soon spread to the Middle Atlantic colonies in the form of academies and private schools; schools flourished to a lesser degree in the South, where tutors provided formal education to the children of plantation owners. The English colonists laid the groundwork for North America's educational system and introduced a variety of sporting activities to the New World. Both of these ingredients were essential for the infusion and development of physical education in U.S. public schools during the nineteenth and twentieth centuries.

AMERICAN INDEPENDENCE AND EUROPEAN INFLUENCES

With American independence, such prominent leaders as Thomas Jefferson, Benjamin Franklin, and Benjamin Rush understood that an educated electorate would best serve the new democracy. Franklin and Jefferson expressed their support for physical activity in their writings about youth and education, while Rush was a prime advocate of education programs for young women.

As the United States began to carve out its own identity during the nineteenth century, it continued to serve as a repository of European ideas and a refuge for European immigrants. Nowhere was this more apparent than in the sphere of education. The educational ideas of Jean-Jacques Rousseau, cultivated and modified by Johann Basedow, Johann Guts Muths, Johann Heinrich Pestalozzi, and Friedrich Jahn, found their way to U.S. shores. They were brought here either by American educators and dignitaries who, on their travels through Europe, observed various educational innovations in operation or by political refugees who sought asylum in America.

Early in the century, Pestalozzian pedagogy, heavily influenced by Rousseau, crossed the Atlantic. Based on Pestalozzi's "object teaching" and learning through the senses (in which physical activity played a crucial role), this movement germinated Pestalozzian schools in Philadelphia as early as 1809 and in New York, Connecticut, Massachusetts, and other states. Its curriculum, which included the natural outdoor activities of running, jumping, and climbing, offered students freedom and opportunities for self-discovery. About the same time, Joseph Lancaster introduced his system of assembly-line education to New York City. The use of

monitors—older pupils who taught lessons in the three R's
and catechism to the younger ones—reduced the cost of instruction, but a prime benefit to students was Lancaster's
recognition of the value of play. Each school had playgrounds, and students could play outside at noon and
throughout the day.[2]

German gymnastics, a third European influence, came to
America during the 1820s, when three disciples of Friedrich
Jahn's turnverein, Charles Beck, Charles Follen, and Fran-
cis Lieber, fled Prussian suppression and migrated to the
Boston area. Beck and Follen arrived in 1824. The following year, Beck found employment as a Latin instructor at
the **Round Hill School** in Northampton, Massachusetts.
Modeled on European boarding schools, this institution was
established in 1823 to improve the cognitive, moral, and
physical faculties of adolescent boys. While at Round Hill,
Beck constructed an outdoor gymnasium and instituted
Jahn's gymnastics, the first program of regular physical
activity in an American curriculum. Beck resigned his position in 1830, two years before the experimental school
closed its doors. He then joined the faculty at Harvard,
where he taught Latin until his retirement.

In 1825 Harvard hired Follen to teach German and devise a gymnastics program for students after Professor John
C. Warren and his colleagues had failed to lure Beck away
from Round Hill or induce Jahn to come to the United
States. During his tenure at Harvard, Follen set up the first
college gymnasium in the United States in 1826 and introduced German gymnastics, which initially attracted a favorable response. In fact, the response was so favorable that
college and city officials established a public gymnasium in
Boston that Follen agreed to supervise until a permanent
superintendent could be hired. At Harvard and the public
gymnasium, Follen employed Lancaster's monitoring
techniques for teaching gymnastics. But enthusiasm for
gymnastics was short-lived, prompting Follen to resign his
position at the Harvard gymnasium in 1828. In 1827 Fran-
cis Lieber took the reins of the public gymnasium after
Jahn declined John Warren's second invitation to come to
Boston. In addition to overseeing the public gymnasium,

Lieber established a swimming school in Boston.[3] By the early 1830s, all of these programs disappeared because they had no means of support, and Americans of the time held a narrow view of physical training for health. The advent of health reform, which formed part of a larger morality crusade, however, caused Americans to expand their view of physical training.

HEALTH AND MORAL REFORM IN THE UNITED STATES

Associated with the United States' growth and development during the early nineteenth century was a widespread health reform movement embedded in a larger moral reform movement that involved antislavery, temperance, women's rights, and Sabbatarianism (observance of the Sabbath). Health reform actually grew out of the temperance movement. Moralists in the 1830s believed that all illness was related to irritations of the gastrointestinal tract caused by poor eating habits or use of alcohol. Sylvester Graham, a Presbyterian minister turned temperance crusader and then health reformer, saw the overstimulation of the digestive tract through improper or excessive eating and ingesting alcohol as threats not only to the human body but also to the Christian soul. Expounding tenets of **Christian physiology,** he proclaimed the virtues of whole-grain bread (the Graham cracker) and a vegetarian diet, moderate food intake, and abstinence from alcohol as antidotes to digestive irritations. He initiated the health reform movement through his lectures and publications, but it was William Alcott who popularized it.[4]

William Alcott—cousin of A. Bronson Alcott, the father of Louisa May—spread the gospel of health reform through his writings, lectures, and teachings. His exposure to Pestalozzian programs as a teacher convinced him of the importance of play and exercise in a child's education. As a schoolmaster, he expressed concern for children's health in his criticism of educational facilities and practices that denied pupils fresh air and physical activity. Graham's ideas gave him the platform he needed to wage his campaign. Like Graham, Alcott was a Christian physiologist who believed

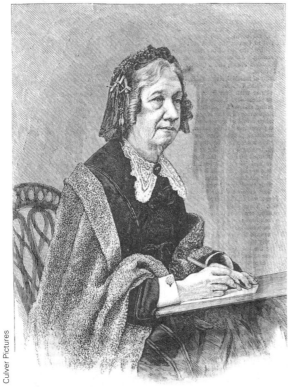

Culver Pictures

Catharine Beecher, pioneer advocate of exercise for women.

that healthful living was part of God's law, for good health not only saved dollars but also saved souls. The combination of exercise, preventive medicine, and Christian principles, Alcott believed, could save American society, and that combination Alcott labeled "Physical Education."[5]

Catharine Beecher, a contemporary of Graham and Alcott, promoted exercise and physical activity for women. The sister of Harriet Beecher Stowe and eldest child of evangelist Lyman Beecher, whose stances on temperance and antislavery thrust him into a leadership position in the moral reform movement, Catharine was a product of Victorian ideology. And as such, she subscribed to the **Cult of True Womanhood,** which wrapped women in a veil of piety, purity, submissiveness, and domesticity. She cast women into subservient roles, not to be subject to men, but to make a better society. She believed exercise would give women strength and stamina to bear healthy children and perform domestic duties.[6]

Like Graham and Alcott, Beecher advocated "Christian physiology," for she, too, believed the unhealthy were inherently immoral. By the 1830s, she had developed calisthenics and exercises for women, based on the Swedish gymnastics of Per Henrik Ling. She campaigned against crowded, stuffy schoolrooms that deprived students of fresh air, and she detested tight corsets and most of the dress of the day, which restricted movement. She also opposed substances (coffee, tea, alcohol, and tobacco) that were detrimental to the body. As an advocate of fresh air and exercise, she favored calisthenics over gymnastics for all children. Gymnastics, she thought, were too strenuous and required special equipment. Her exercises, as outlined in her *Physiology and Calisthenics for Schools and Families* (1856) and elsewhere, could be done virtually anywhere. A lifelong educator with a strong belief in education for women, she founded female seminaries in Hartford, Connecticut, in 1824, and Cincinnati, Ohio, in 1833. Her firm commitment to bring women into teaching led her to establish an organization that sent 450 teachers to Indiana, Illinois, Iowa, Wisconsin, and several other Western states from 1847 to 1857. But Beecher was not alone in creating educational institutions for women. Emma Willard and Mary Lyon founded the Troy Female Seminary (1821) and Mount Holyoke Female Seminary (1837), respectively. Their programs, similar to Beecher's, emphasized domesticity and included exercise and calisthenics to preserve the health of young women.[7]

Sharing the views of Beecher, Willard, and Lyon was Elizabeth Blackwell, the first female physician in the United States. She believed that women should be strong to carry out their childbearing and child-rearing roles. Her vision of human nature, however, extended far beyond the realm of natural and domestic duties ascribed to women. From a much broader perspective, contained in her *Laws of Life*, Blackwell viewed the human body as *Divine Humanity*. Forging tenets of Christian physiology with her own view of humankind, she believed a healthy body was the precursor to a healthy mind and soul, and exercise was the fundamental law upon which the others were built. Exercise, in her view, enabled one to grow as it prepared one for life. Once the body was developed through vigorous exercise, the development of the mind and soul would follow. She called for vigorous exercise until the age of puberty, then nourishment for the mind and soul, which needed more attention during adulthood. Even though the body needed less attention during adulthood, it was not to be neglected. In Blackwell's schema, humankind can "accomplish [its] own happiness and fulfill the idea of creation."[8]

As the health reform movement continued to attract followers, enterprising opportunists with monetary motives jumped on the bandwagon. One such opportunist was Dioclesian ("Dio") Lewis, whose ill health or hypochondria led him to study medicine at Harvard and then homeopathy, a practice of preventing disease in a healthy person by creating its symptoms. Ultimately, his interest in preventive medicine led him to discover exercise and calisthenics, from which he devised what he called "the New Gymnastics." This form of light exercise was done individually or in pairs with bean bags, wands, rings, dumbbells, and Indian clubs. Lewis reacted to the heavy exercises promoted by George Barker Windship and other strength-seekers of the period. Both Lewis and Windship believed physical exercise was a necessary prerequisite to sound health, but they differed on the approach. Windship held that strength, through heavy lifting, was the key, whereas Lewis advocated light, free-flowing exercises that required only a modicum of strength. An itinerant and captivating speaker, Lewis touted "New Gymnastics" for public schools, but he emerged in the public spotlight following his lecture on "The New System of Gymnastics" at the 1860 Boston convention of the American Institute for Instruction. The convention endorsed his program and urged public schools to adopt it. As his reputation grew, Lewis attracted enough public support to publish a journal and open the Normal Institute for Physical Education in Boston. From 1861 to 1868, his normal school produced 250 graduates. The Civil War sparked renewed interest in military drill, which eventually eclipsed gymnastics as the favored mode of exercise for youth, causing Lewis to shut down his school in 1868. Nevertheless, he continued to preach "New Gymnastics" well into his later years.[9]

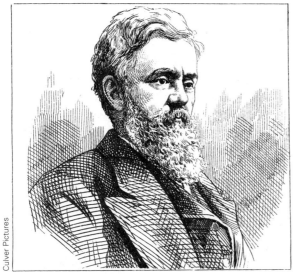

Dio Lewis designed "New Gymnastics" for people of all ages.

As the United States' cities grew and expanded during the middle decades of the nineteenth century, saloons, gambling halls, and brothels, by-products of urban expansion, increased in number. Those seedbeds of vice, as moralists labeled them, tempted youth, particularly young men, and threatened their moral integrity. The Young Men's Christian Association, imported from England by George Petrie in 1852, offered programs that moralists believed would counter the unsavory behavior associated with drinking, gambling, or prostitution. Initially YMCAs provided reading rooms where young men might read local newspapers, participate in Bible study, or engage in conversation with others; but after the Civil War the YMCAs constructed gymnasiums and later swimming pools and other facilities in order to keep young men occupied through physical activity. After the first gymnasiums appeared in 1869 in New York City and San Francisco, this trend spread to cities across America, leading to the opening of 348 gymnasiums by 1891. At first, circus performers, prize fighters, and professional athletes directed physical activity programs at the Ys because no formal professional preparation programs existed. This condition changed and the quality of instruction improved after 1887 with the establishment of the YMCA Training School at Springfield, Massachusetts.[10]

The female counterpart of the YMCA movement, the YWCA, appeared in 1866. It provided single women with living quarters and recreational outlets. By the 1880s its health-conscious programs included calisthenics and exercise.[11]

In the postbellum United States, three health crusaders—Horace Fletcher, John Harvey Kellogg, and Bernarr Macfadden—continued to fan the flames of reform. All three believed in a vegetarian diet, though Macfadden was not completely opposed to eating flesh, and his open glorification of sexuality was a departure from orthodox **Victorian era** beliefs held by the other two. Fletcher supported mastication, or endless chewing, until all taste was gone in order to reduce appetite and enhance digestion. Kellogg, borrowing from Graham and Fletcher, established a sanitarium in Battle Creek, Michigan, that provided vegetarian meals, hydropathy (hot and cold water treatments), and other therapeutic remedies for physical ailments. Macfadden, a fitness guru who saw "weakness as a crime," considered exercise the supreme elixir for virility, the bedrock of good health. Diet, fresh air, sunshine, and cleanliness combined with exercise purified the blood and prevented disease, but exercise was by far the most important component. Macfadden turned fitness and health reform into a multimillion-dollar business, mostly through the publication *Physical Culture* and several confession-type magazines. Medical professionals and physical educators, most of whom were physicians, derided him as a charlatan, chiefly because he recommended exercise and fasting over drugs and standard medical treatments to combat illness.[12] In spite of the criticism, as the nineteenth century drew to a close, Macfadden's efforts kept before the public the message of health reform and the value of exercise, initiated some seventy years earlier.

GYMNASTICS, GERMANS, AND THE TURNVEREIN

Another force that imprinted the value of exercise on the American mind was the influx of German immigrants, who fled political upheaval and instability in Prussia and other German states and came to the United States during the first half of the nineteenth century. Though immigrants arrived in waves, one of the largest groups came following uprisings in 1848. Some "forty-eighters," as they were called, settled in cities on the East Coast, but a majority booked passage on Southern cotton boats that otherwise would have returned empty. They entered the country via New Orleans and traveled up the Mississippi River and its tributaries to St. Louis, Louisville, Cincinnati, Kansas City, Chicago, Milwaukee, and other midwestern cities. Germans, like most immigrant groups, brought their customs and traditions with them. Beer gardens, songfests, and the turnverein were commonplace in German neighborhoods. The popularity of **turner** societies, with their emphasis on gymnastics and other forms of physical activity, led to the formation of the **North American turnerbund.** The bund sponsored annual turnfests in which representatives from the turner societies gathered each year to demonstrate their athletic and martial skills and display their native German customs.[13]

The Civil War disrupted turnverein activities as large numbers of forty-eighters enlisted in the Union and Confederate armies. But the return of peace in 1865 saw Germans revive their turner societies. They reestablished turnfests and in 1866 opened the Normal School of the North American Gymnastics Union in New York City to train gymnastics instructors for the turner clubs. The Normal School moved to Chicago in 1870, then to Milwaukee, and finally to Indianapolis. After their arrival in the United States, but particularly following the Civil War, German turners not only promoted gymnastics for the public schools but also pressed for compulsory physical education laws. In 1885, through the influence of Carl Betz, Kansas City's school district was the first to adopt gymnastics. Ten other midwestern cities soon followed suit, giving German gymnastics a stronghold in the West.[14] The East, however, was quite a different story.

SWEDISH GYMNASTICS AND THE BATTLE OF THE SYSTEMS

Elements of Per Henrik Ling's system of gymnastics had been adopted prior to the Civil War by both Catharine Beecher and Dio Lewis for their exercise and calisthenics programs; but in the 1880s Swedish gymnastics molded its own identity. Hartvig Nissen, vice-consul of Norway and Sweden, began teaching Swedish gymnastics to a group of teachers and students in Washington, D.C., in 1883, and to students at Johns Hopkins in 1887. In 1885 Nissen received a visit from Baron Nils Posse, a Swedish nobleman with a commendable military record and a recent graduate of Ling's gymnastics institute.

Anxious to establish his own practice of medical gymnastics, Posse settled in Boston, hoping to find support for his program from the medical profession in that city. Unable to attract physician support, he found a constituency, quite fortuitously, for his program in the Boston public schools. When Mary Hemenway, a philanthropist who had been

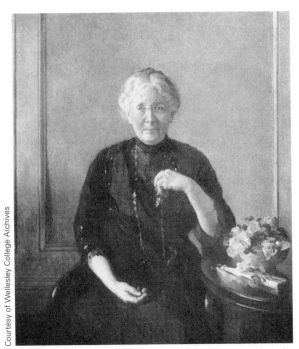

Courtesy of Wellesley College Archives

Amy Morris Homans molded female physical educators for some thirty years.

providing programs in domestic crafts for Boston schoolchildren, realized that youth needed physical training, a friend put her in contact with Posse. Impressed with his program, she quickly brought Posse under her employ and then extended an offer of one year's free training to 100 Boston teachers, if the school district would adopt Swedish gymnastics for its pupils. This experiment, with Posse preparing public school teachers to teach gymnastics, was highly successful. By 1890 the Boston School District institutionalized Swedish gymnastics and then summoned Edward Hartwell to serve as director of physical training, a position he held until 1897. Nissen served as Hartwell's assistant and then succeeded him as director from 1897 to 1900.[15]

One significant outgrowth of the Boston experiment in Swedish gymnastics was the formation of the **Boston Normal School of Gymnastics.** Established by Hemenway, the school functioned for twenty years under the direction of Amy Morris Homans, the founder's long-time secretary, before amalgamating with Wellesley College in 1909. Homans continued to administer the program at Wellesley until her retirement in 1919. During her thirty-year tenure, her program prepared more than 600 young women to teach gymnastics and physical education.[16]

Hemenway's interest in the Swedish system led her in 1889 to finance the **Boston Conference on Physical Training,** which attracted more than 2,000 people. Chaired by U.S. Commissioner of Education William T. Harris, the conference, in extolling the benefits of physical training, provided an open forum to settle the **Battle of the Systems** through discussion of German, Swedish, and other gymnastics systems in use. Although the conference attracted considerable interest in the various systems of gymnastics, its impact was short-lived as sports, games, and natural activities began to replace gymnastics as the preferred activities of the physical education curriculum.[17]

THE GERMINATION OF PHYSICAL EDUCATION AS A PROFESSION

Simultaneously with the influences of Swedish and German gymnastics on physical training in America, Edward Hitchcock at Amherst, Dudley Sargent at Harvard, William Anderson at Adelphi and Yale, and Delphine Hanna at Oberlin College began laying the groundwork for formalized instruction in physical education at their respective institutions. Hitchcock, Sargent, and Anderson used anthropometric measurement to establish norms for college men in order to determine their physical activity needs, while Hanna measured college women for similar reasons. They all saw the need for required physical education for college students and developed exercise programs by borrowing from the Swedish and German systems, Dio Lewis, François Delsarte (light, muscle flexibility routines combined with elocution exercises) and other forms of gymnastics training. They then modified them to suit their own beliefs and practices.

Hitchcock took over physical training at Amherst in 1861 and spent nearly fifty years there promoting physical education. Sargent began his career as a circus performer, but then received a M.D. from Yale before operating a private gymnasium in New York City. When Harvard constructed a new gymnasium in 1879 with Hemenway money, Sargent, on the recommendation of Harvard alumnus and former crew coach William Blaikie, was hired. He devised more than forty exercise machines and established the Harvard Summer School for the preparation of physical education teachers. By 1904 he had trained 261 teachers; some reports credit his summer school courses with attracting more than 5,000 teachers during his forty years at Harvard. Sargent and Hitchcock were instrumental in the 1885 meeting called by William G. Anderson of Adelphi College, which attracted physicians, gymnasium directors, and others involved in the instruction of physical activity. Anderson, who had observed great variation among physical education programs, including disparate gymnastics systems, organized this meeting to bring some continuity to physical education instruction. Though that did not happen, his efforts led to the formation of the **Association for the Advancement of Physical Education (AAPE)—** currently, American Alliance for Health, Physical Education, Recreation and Dance (AAHPERD). Edward Hitchcock was elected the new organization's first president.[18]

Hitchcock's election, no doubt, was a tribute to his many contributions, particularly his recognition as the founder of college physical education programs. At Amherst, Hitchcock instituted anthropometry and is credited with being the first American to apply **anthropometric measurement** to physical education programs. After taking and tabulating thousands of student measurements over a twenty-five-year period, he concluded that height was the best predictor of various body proportions. Based on the "average" college student's height of 67.9 inches, he devised an "Average Anthropometric Table" that enabled him to identify "average" body measurements for chest girth, arm girth, lung capacity, and other physical parameters of every college student.[19]

Sargent, too, conducted anthropometric measurements, but his purpose was "to improve the physical condition of the mass of students" and to identify those in greatest need of physical training. He then prescribed individual exercise regimens, which he believed would "enable them to perform the duties that await them after leaving college." The uniqueness of his program lay in the exercise apparatus and devices he developed with weights and pulleys that students could adjust to meet his individual needs. Under Sargent's direction, more than 50,000 physical examinations were conducted in his department. Though no promoter of intercollegiate athletics, Sargent insisted, for safety reasons, that students undergo strength testing in order to qualify for athletic teams. The criteria for football and crew were the highest.[20]

Having studied under Sargent, Dio Lewis, and Nils Posse, Delphine Hanna adopted gymnastic exercises for her program at Oberlin College, though her focus, possibly due to

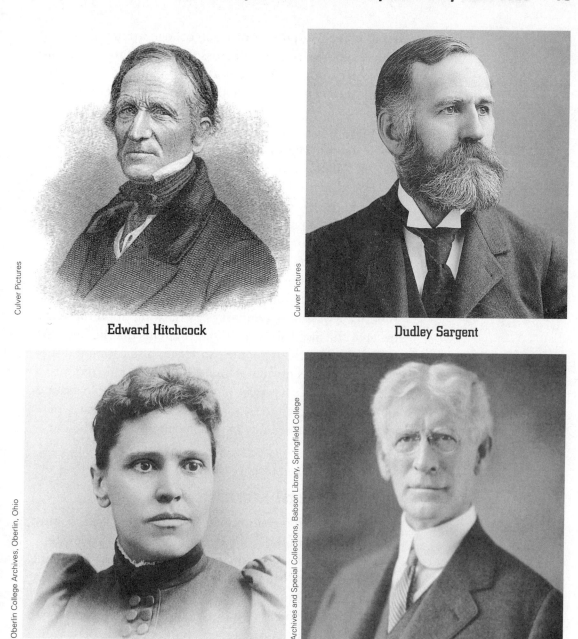

Culver Pictures

Edward Hitchcock

Culver Pictures

Dudley Sargent

Oberlin College Archives, Oberlin, Ohio

Delphine Hanna

Archives and Special Collections, Babson Library, Springfield College

William Anderson

Four pioneers who shaped physical education into a profession.

Sargent's influence, turned toward orthopedics and remedial exercises. She believed that the gymnasium teacher should use gymnastics to treat postural deformities and physical ailments. She developed an anthropometric chart based on measurements of 1,600 college women that female physical educators across the country used to compare their students' anatomical and physiological features so that they could prescribe the appropriate exercises. Hanna's legacy, though, is embedded in the prominent professionals she taught and guided at Oberlin—Thomas Wood, Luther Halsey Gulick, Fred Eugene Leonard, Jesse Feiring Williams, Jay B. Nash, and Gertrude Moulton, who succeeded her at Oberlin.[21]

Like Hanna and Sargent, William G. Anderson had a great interest in teacher training. He opened normal schools at Adelphi and New Haven, Connecticut, and founded the Chautauqua Summer School, which had a reputation for teacher training second only to Sargent's summer program at Harvard. Anderson attempted to devise an American system of gymnastics by drawing upon those aspects of the Swedish and German systems that he believed suited the American people. Anderson also promoted specialization at his normal schools. Believing that students could not master all styles of gymnastics, he employed specialists in each area to expose his students to a variety of styles with the possibility of specializing in one if they so desired.[22]

INTERCOLLEGIATE ATHLETICS

Concurrent with developments in physical education, athletics emerged in the colleges and universities. Following the Revolutionary War and in the early decades of the nineteenth century, a college education was accessible only to a privileged few; but as the United States grew and expanded due to the twin forces of industrialization and technology, a newly rich social class emerged, built on an aristocracy of wealth. Self-made businessmen, who mostly constituted this class, now had the financial resources to send their sons off to the university; and this new breed of college student rebelled against colleges' strict authoritarian regulations and their classical curriculum of Latin, Greek, and theology. Some reaction was negative: Students disrupted chapel services, pulled pranks on professors, and engaged in riotous behavior that caused injury and property damage. Positive responses led to the creation of the extracurriculum. First to appear were literary societies and debate teams, followed by fraternities, and then athletics, arguably the extracurriculum's most prominent component.

College athletics actually emerged from class rushes, an initiation rite at Harvard, Yale, and other institutions, in which freshmen were pitted against upperclassmen in a football (actually soccer) game. With merely one ball and twenty-five to thirty on a side, the contest quickly turned into a morass of bloody noses and bruised shins. These rushes created a camaraderie that led to the formation of sporting clubs on campus, the necessary structure for intercollegiate competition. By the fifth decade of the nineteenth century, students at both Harvard and Yale organized rowing clubs. One entrepreneur, James N. Elkins of the Boston, Concord and Montreal Railroad, saw an opportunity to enhance his rail operation and entice Bostonians to purchase vacation property on Lake Winnipesaukee, New Hampshire. In 1852 he invited the rowing clubs at both universities to an eight-day, expenses-paid holiday on the New Hampshire lake, if they would race each other at the end of their stay. They agreed, and the race won by Harvard ushered in intercollegiate athletics in America.[23] Soon afterward, intercollegiate competition began in baseball (1859), cricket (1864), and football (1869).

Although crew was the dominant sport in the early history of college athletics, football, by the end of the century, reigned king—evolving from soccer to rugby and then to American football. The first intercollegiate football game played between Princeton and Rutgers was actually a game of soccer that Rutgers won, 6–4. In the early 1870s students at McGill University in Montreal introduced their Harvard counterparts to rugby, which the Americans liked better than soccer. Rugby then caught the eye of college students elsewhere and became the football game of choice on college campuses. During the 1880s Walter Camp emerged as a player and then coach at Yale. He gained a decisive position on the Rules Committee, which enabled him to play a crucial role in the transformation of rugby into American football. He converted the heel-out rugby scrum into the line of scrimmage with a center snap. Later rules changes would set seven men on the line of scrimmage, modify the scoring system, and designate specific duties for blockers and runners.[24]

Initially students controlled intercollegiate athletics. Their lack of business and administrative acumen often put their institutions in debt, and their exuberance for winning, sometimes unfairly with brutal and unethical play, raised the ire of the faculty and college officials. In the mid-1880s Harvard faculty members established an Athletic Committee to oversee athletics and reduce, if not eliminate, student control. And with creditors knocking on their door, college presidents supported their faculty's efforts to regulate athletic finances. But they also saw athletics as an advertising medium that increased the visibility of their institution, attracted students, and fostered the concept of alma mater among alumni. Realizing the economic benefits of athletics, presidents wanted their intercollegiate programs to survive, but with certain controls.[25]

Faculty and administrative control harnessed spending on athletics, but it could not control behavior on the playing field. During the 1890s and early 1900s, brutal play led to a number of deaths. Some colleges like Columbia, Northwestern, and Stanford dropped football; others were ready to follow suit. It took a strong effort by Harvard, Yale, and others dedicated to football to reform the game and keep it going. The dire situation reached a climax in 1905, when twelve deaths from brutality on the football field led the reformers to take action and create the NCAA. This organization, which became the governing body of collegiate athletics in 1906, modified the rules to reduce deaths and head injuries. It created a more open game that permitted the forward pass and extended the yardage necessary for a first down from five to ten yards.[26]

While football underwent metamorphosis, a new game, basketball, appeared on the collegiate landscape in 1891. James Naismith, under the direction of Luther Gulick at the YMCA Training School in Springfield, Massachusetts, devised this game to keep students occupied during the

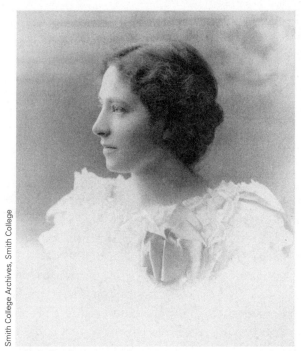

Senda Berenson devised basketball rules for women.

winter months between the fall and spring sport seasons. As the game caught on, both men and women played it, but women took to it on the intercollegiate level more quickly than did men. Senda Berenson of Smith College modified rules for the women's game during the 1890s. She divided the court into three zones and placed nine women on a team, with three players per team restricted to each zone. She was, of course, reacting to the dictates of Victorian ideology, which held that excessive physical activity, such as running the length of a basketball court, would damage women's childbearing organs. Nevertheless, in spite of Victorian mores, some nineteenth-century college women participated in archery, baseball, rowing, tennis, and track, with Vassar and Smith Colleges leading the way.[27]

AMATEUR ATHLETICS AND THE REVIVAL OF THE OLYMPIC GAMES

Outside the confines of educational institutions, athletics also prospered during the latter half of the nineteenth century. Like college sports, they germinated in club settings, either in neighborhoods and the workplace, where baseball and cricket emerged, or in metropolitan athletic clubs, where track and field, wrestling, cycling, swimming, and football crystallized. In these venues an amateur spirit prevailed until the importance of winning superseded the joy of participation; this happened quickly in baseball and football. Baseball turned professional within twenty-five years of the introduction of the New York Game (the current version of baseball with a few modifications) in 1846; football began to convert to professionalism in 1892, almost immediately after surfacing in athletic clubs. Track and field, apart from pedestrian marathon races, remained amateur and became the core events of the modern Olympic Games, revived in 1896.

The modern games, designed to foster harmony among the nations of the world, grew out of nineteenth-century European nationalism. Early in the century, Napoleon's military success against Prussia and his aggrandizement of Europe caused German nationalists to organize the turn-verein in order to strengthen youth for military purposes. By the 1870s, Prussia had the strongest army on the continent, which prevailed in the Franco-Prussian War, costing France valuable territory. Among the land ceded to Prussia was a parcel that a young French noble, Baron Pierre de Coubertin, stood to inherit upon his father's death. Partly because of the lost territory and partly because of France's inept performance against the Prussian army, Coubertin wanted a strong and secure France, a motherland that generated pride amongst her citizens. His readings and travels, especially to England, exposed him to the Olympic Games of the ancient Greeks. The resurrection of the Olympics, he believed, would stimulate France to initiate a broad-based national sports program to identify and train potential competitors. A sports program and training regimen of nationwide magnitude would reach the masses of French youth, and ultimately this process would produce stronger young men for the French army. Coubertin set out to revive the Games, but, contrary to popular belief, he was not solely responsible for their rebirth.[28]

Greek nationalists Panagiotis Soutsos and Evangelis Zappas and British physician William Penny Brookes played significant roles in reinstating the Games. Soutsos, a Greek patriot, expressed his sentiment for Greek nationalism in his poetry as early as 1833. He called upon the Greeks to reinstate the Games with the intent of returning Greece to its former glory. He even petitioned the Greek government to revive the Games, though his plea ultimately fell upon deaf ears. But in the 1850s Evangelis Zappas took up Soutsos's cause. He left 200,000 drachmas to the Greek government to renovate the stadium at Athens and to prepare facilities for athletic contests to be held in 1859.

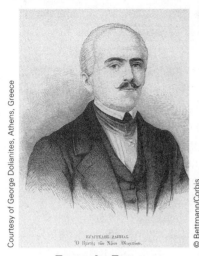 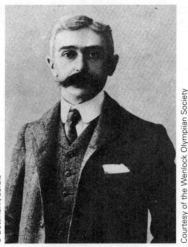 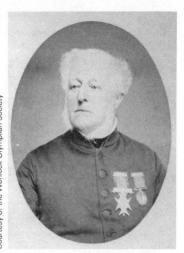

Evangelis Zappas   **Pierre de Coubertin**   **William Penny Brooks**

These three men played significant roles in the revival of the Olympic Games.

Meanwhile in England, in 1850 Dr. Brookes organized the Wenlock Olympian Games as part of his program to help farmers and the working class to improve themselves; he also established a reading society for them. Learning about the Zappas proposal from the newspaper, Brookes contacted the Greek government and suggested several events that might be included in the games. On the home front, Brookes's Olympic Games expanded to regional and even international competitions, held in London in 1866. When in the late 1880s Coubertin discovered the speech Brookes gave on physical degeneracy prior to the London Olympics, he contacted Brookes and made arrangements to visit him in 1890. During the visit, Brookes reenacted his annual Olympic Games for Coubertin, giving the visitor the idea to restore the Games from ancient Greece. With Coubertin's effort and the support of the Greek government, the modern Olympic Games were reborn at Athens in 1896. The Games may not have been revived without the French baron's drive and perseverance, but credit for the revival is not Coubertin's alone.[29]

At the first modern Games, Americans excelled, winning nine of the twelve championships in track and field. In fact, the United States did not even send its best athletes who, at that time affiliated with the New York Athletic Club, showed no interest in participating in the Olympic Games. Ten athletes from Princeton University and the Boston Athletic Association formed the U.S. team. They trained, for the most part, on shipboard during their journey to Athens. Arriving just one day before the competition began, the Americans, with little time to acclimate, nevertheless performed well. James Connolly won the triple jump and became the first American to win an Olympic championship as well as the first Olympic victor in the modern Games.[30]

As the nineteenth century drew to a close, Americans demonstrated their penchant for athletics on both the amateur and professional levels. Intercollegiate athletic programs emerged and expanded, while baseball set the pace among the professional ranks, with other sports moving in that direction. Physical education had established itself as a legitimate profession, having evolved from the health and moral reform movement with influences from German and Swedish gymnastics. Physical education and athletics, both professional and amateur, were on solid footing to meet the challenges of the twentieth century.

On the Web

www.aafla.org
Web site of the Amateur Athletic Federation of Los Angeles, which is a storehouse of information on the modern Olympic Games. It also has online issues of the *Journal of Sport History, Journal of Olympic History, Olympika, International Sports Studies, Iron Game History, and Outing.*

www.olympic.org
Official Web site of Olympic movement; has capsule summaries of the summer and winter games of each Olympiad from 1896.

http://www.fhw.gr/projects/olympics
Web site of the Foundation of the Hellenic World; contains good information on the ancient and modern Olympic games.

http://schools.eastnet.ecu.edu/pitt/ayden/hist/history.html
Web site at Ayden Elementary School that has photos and brief description of early leaders in physical education, such as Beecher, Lewis, Beck, and Follen.

http://encarta.msn.com/encnet/refpages/RefArticle.aspx?refid=
761560297&pn=1#s2
Encyclopedia article that contains information on the history of physical
education.

Key Terms

anthropometric measurement Bodily measurements (height, weight,
arm, chest, waist girth, and the like) taken by Edward Hitchcock, Dudley
Sargent, Delphine Hanna, and other early physical educators to develop
norms and classify college students (page 74).

Association for the Advancement of Physical Education (AAPE) Original name of AAHPERD, founded in 1885 as an outgrowth of a meeting
of physicians, gymnasium directors, and others involved in the instruction of physical activity (page 74).

Battle of the Systems Debate between the proponents of German and
Swedish gymnastics over the merits of each system (page 72).

Boston Conference on Physical Training Conference in 1889 financed
by Mary Hemenway to provide an open forum for the discussion of German, Swedish, and other gymnastics systems in use. It was chaired by
U.S. Commissioner of Education William T. Harris and attracted more
than 2,000 people (page 72).

Boston Normal School of Gymnastics Founded and financed by Mary
Hemenway and headed by Amy Morris Homans for the preparation of
young women to teach Swedish gymnastics. It was an outgrowth of the
Swedish-German gymnastics debate (page 72).

Christian physiology An early-nineteenth-century belief and moral
standard promoted by Sylvester Graham and William Alcott; it viewed
all bodily ailments as gastrointestinal, caused by improper diet and imbibing alcohol. An ailing body, in turn, damaged the soul (page 65).

court ball Rigorous ball game played by Aztec and Mayan Indians on an
I-shaped court. Objective was to propel a softball-sized rubber ball
through a ring without using the hands or feet (page 60).

Cult of True Womanhood Nineteenth-century conception of the traits
and characteristics an upper- and middle-class woman should possess—
piety, purity, submissiveness, and domesticity (page 66).

lacrosse North American Indians played this game of dexterity in which
sticks with small baskets were used to catch and propel a small ball into a
small goal (page 60).

Round Hill School Early boarding school in Northampton, Massachusetts, designed to improve the cognitive, moral, and physical attributes
of adolescent boys. Charles Beck introduced Jahn's gymnastics there,

making it the first program of regular physical activity in an American curriculum (page 64).

North American turnerbund Organization of German turner societies in North America that sponsored annual festivals, turnfests, and other functions (page 70).

ring tourney Popular activity in Southern states in which a horse rider at full gallop attempted to insert his lance into a small suspended ring (page 62).

shinny Game, similar to modern field hockey, played by North American Indians (page 60).

turners German immigrants who brought to America their system of gymnastics, which they learned as members of the turnverein in Prussia and other German states (page 70).

Victorian era Period of history throughout most of the nineteenth century that mirrored the reign of Queen Victoria in England, 1837–1901 (page 69).

Multiple Choice Questions

1. German gymnastics received great impetus in the United States from German organizations called

   a. sokols
   b. falcons
   c. turners
   d. moonies
   e. none of the above

2. The European influences on American education and physical education were

   a. German turners
   b. Lancastrian system
   c. Pestalozzian movement
   d. a and b of the above
   e. a, b and c of the above

3. The first American school to make gymnastics a part of the school program was

   a. Latin Grammar School
   b. Harvard University
   c. Round Hill School
   d. Amherst College
   e. Franklin's Academy

4. The French baron involved in the revival of the Olympic Games was

   a. Pierre de Coubertin
   b. Marquis de Lafayette
   c. Jean-Jacques Rousseau

    d. Tom Brown

    e. Alexis de Tocqueville

5. The person who used Graham's platform to popularize the health reform movement along with popularizing the Pestalozzian Movement in America was

    a. Sylvester Graham

    b. William Alcott

    c. Bernarr Macfadden

    d. Horace Fletcher

    e. John H. Kellogg

6. The secretary to Mary Hemenway who directed the Boston Normal School of Gymnastics was

    a. Senda Berenson

    b. Amy Morris Homans

    c. Delphine Hanna

    d. Edward Hartwell

    e. Dudley Sargent

7. The philanthropist who financed the introduction of Swedish gymnastics in the Boston public schools was

    a. Nils Posse

    b. Amy Morris Homans

    c. Edward Hartwell

    d. Hartvig Nissen

    e. Mary Hemenway

8. The outcome of the 1885 meeting of physical directors summoned by William G. Anderson was the

    a. end of the Battle of the Systems

    b. founding of Boston Normal School

    c. formation of AAHPERD

    d. demise of German turnverein

    e. none of the above

9. Piety, purity, submissiveness, and domesticity were the four cardinal virtues of

    a. robust manliness

    b. ghost busters

    c. the feminist movement

    d. the feminine mystique

    e. the cult of true womanhood

10. Anthropometric measurements of physical parameters (height, weight, chest girth, arm girth, and the like) were used to classify college students by

    a. Edward Hitchcock

    b. Dudley Sargent
    c. Delphine Hanna
    d. a and b of the above
    e. a, b, and c of the above

Critical Thinking Questions

1. The Health Reform Movement of the nineteenth century was tied closely to morality and moral reform. Why were health and morals bonded together, and how did this relationship contribute to the emergence of physical education?

2. Catharine Beecher was in the forefront of promoting education for young women, yet she believed in the Cult of True Womanhood, which may appear to us as a contradiction in values and gender equity. What accounts for Beecher's seemingly contradictory value structure, and why would the Cult of True Womanhood be acceptable in the nineteenth century and not today?

3. From the meticulous research of David Young, we know that the Greeks and English, in addition to the Frenchman Pierre de Coubertin, played prominent roles in the revival of the Olympic Games in 1896. Even though Coubertin interacted with both the Greeks and English in his quest to bring the games back, he always promoted himself as the sole author of the Olympic revival. Why did he deliberately overlook the Greek and British contributions?

4. You are a school principal in the 1880s who has just returned from the Boston Conference of 1889, where you have heard advocates of both German and Swedish gymnastics discuss the merits and shortcomings of each system. On the basis of what you heard, which system would you adopt for your school and why?

5. Intercollegiate athletics emerged from the extracurriculum and were created by students. With all the problems related to athletics (brutality, cheating, missing classes, gambling, and so on), why did most college presidents throw their support behind intercollegiate athletics on their campuses?

References

1. Allen Guttmann, "Puritans at Play? Accusations and Replies," in *A Whole New Ball Game: An Interpretation of American Sports* (Chapel Hill, N.C.: University of North Carolina Press, 1988), 17–32; J. Thomas Jable, "The English Puritans: Suppressors of Sport and Amusement?" *Canadian Journal of History of Sport and Physical Education*, 7, no. 1 (May 1976): 33–40; Nancy Struna, "Puritans and Sport: The Irretrievable Tide of Change," *Journal of Sport History*, 4, no. 1 (Spring 1977): 1–21;

Foster Rhea Dulles, *A History of Recreation: America Learns to Play,* 2d ed. (New York: Appleton-Century-Crofts, 1965), 3–21.

2. Deobold B. Van Dalen and Bruce L. Bennett, *A World History of Physical Education,* 2d ed. (Englewood Cliffs, N.J.: Prentice-Hall, 1971), 372–73; Arthur Weston, *The Making of American Physical Education* (New York: Appleton-Century-Crofts, 1962), 10–12.

3. Erich Geldbach, "The Beginning of German Gymnastics in America," *Journal of Sport History,* 3, no. 3 (Winter 1976): 236–72; Bruce L. Bennett, "The Making of Round Hill School," *Quest Monograph,* 4 (April 1965): 53–64.

4. Harvy Green, *Fit for America: Health, Fitness and Sport in American Society* (Baltimore: Johns Hopkins University Press, 1986), 45–53; Richard H. Shryock, "Sylvester Graham and the Popular Health Movement, 1830–1870," *Mississippi Valley Historical Review,* 18 (September 1931): 172–83.

5. Green, 27–28.

6. Kathryn Kish Sklar, *Catharine Beecher: A Study in American Domesticity* (New Haven: Yale University Press, 1973), 151–67.

7. Catharine E. Beecher, *Physiology and Calisthenics for Schools and Families* (New York: Harper & Brothers, 1856); Linda J. Borish, "The Robust Woman and the Muscular Christian: Catharine Beecher, Thomas Higginson, and Their Vision of American Society, Health, and Physical Activities," *International Journal of History of Sport,* 4, no. 2 (September 1987): 139–53.

8. Elizabeth Blackwell, *The Laws of Life, with Special Reference to the Physical Education of Girls* (New York: George P. Putnam, 1852).

9. Green, 184–91; Joan Paul, "The Health Reformers: George Barker Windship and Boston's Strength Seekers," *Journal of Sport History,* 10, no. 3 (Winter 1983): 41–57.

10. Van Dalen and Bennett, 411–12.

11. Weston, 45.

12. James C. Whorton, *Crusaders for Fitness: The History of American Health Reformers* (Princeton: Princeton University Press, 1982), 168–238; Robert Ernst, *Weakness Is a Crime: The Life of Bernarr Macfadden* (Syracuse: Syracuse University Press, 1991).

13. Robert K. Barney, "Forty-Eighters and the Rise of the Turnverein Movement in America," in *Ethnicity and Sport in North American History and Culture,* ed. George Eisen and David Wiggins (Westport, Conn.: Greenwood Press, 1994), 19–42.

14. Robert K. Barney, "German Turners in America: Their Role in Nineteenth Century Exercise Expression and Physical Education Legislation," in *A History of Physical Education and Sport in the United States and Canada,* ed. Earle F. Zeigler (Champaign, Ill.: Stipes, 1975), 111–20.

15. Weston, 35; Ellen W. Gerber, *Innovations and Institutions in Physical Education* (Philadelphia: Lea & Febiger, 1971), pp. 308–18.

16. Gerber, p. 313.

17. Weston, 37–39.

18. Gerber, 332–38.

19. Ibid., 280–81.

20. Ibid., 283–91.

21. Ibid., 325–31; Fredrick D. Shults, "Oberlin College: Molder of Four Great Men." *Quest Monograph,* 11 (December 1968): 71–75.

22. Gerber, 332–38.

23. Guy M. Lewis, "Sport and the Making of American Higher Education: The Early Years, 1783–1875," *73rd Proceedings, National College Physical Education Association for Men* (December 23–30, 1970): 208–13; Ronald A. Smith, *Sports and Freedom: The Rise of Big-Time College Athletics* (New York: Oxford University Press, 1988), 13–35.

24. John A. Lucas and Ronald A. Smith, *Saga of American Sport* (Philadelphia: Lea & Febiger, 1978), 229–47; Smith, *Sport and Freedom,* 83–88.

25. Lucas and Smith, 210–26.

26. Smith, 191–208.

27. Senda Berenson, "Significance of Basketball for Women," *Line Basketball for Women,* ed. Senda Berenson (New York: A. G. Spalding, 1901); Betty Spears and Richard A. Swanson, *History of Sport and Physical Education in the United States,* 3d ed. (Dubuque, Iowa: Wm. C. Brown, 1988), pp. 141–45.

28. David C. Young, *The Modern Olympics: A Struggle for Revival* (Baltimore: Johns Hopkins University Press, 1996), 68–80.

29. Ibid., 1–53.

30. Richard D. Mandell, *The First Modern Olympics* (Berkeley: University of California Press, 1976), 123–51.

5

PHYSICAL EDUCATION AND SPORT
IN THE TWENTIETH CENTURY

Chapter Objectives

After reading this chapter, the student will be able to

- Define the "new physical education" and identify at least three of its proponents

- Describe the emergence of interscholastic athletics and their relationship to physical education

- Explain the rationale behind the "athletics are educational" doctrine

- Identify and interpret at least three contributing forces to compulsory state physical education legislation

- Describe and compare the participation and competition models of women's sports during the 1920s

- Describe the outcome of the fitness explosion triggered by the Kraus-Weber tests

PROGRESSIVISM AND PROGRESSIVE EDUCATION IN THE NEW CENTURY

Although rooted in the nineteenth century, **Progressivism** blossomed in the twentieth. Sparked by the spirit of reform emanating from the Populist movement in rural states and the debilitating, squalid living conditions of urban environments, Progressivism produced significant changes in government, agriculture, banking, business, social services, housing, and education. The Progressive movement brought about the direct election of senators, the Federal Reserve System, federal income tax, antitrust legislation, the Food and Drug Administration, urban sanitation, and improved housing and living conditions. During the closing decades of the nineteenth century, this ideology spilled over into the **progressive education** movement and then to physical education.

G. Stanley Hall's monumental work on child development, *Adolescence,* caused educators to begin looking at learning from a different perspective. Curriculum focused on the child, whose maturation level determined learning. Edward Thorndike and William James adopted and promulgated Hall's ideas on educating youth. Then John Dewey, the most prominent progressive educator, instituted the child-centered curriculum not only to facilitate students' learning but also to prepare them to function effectively in a democratic society. At his demonstration schools in Chicago and later at Columbia University, he applied Hall's and James's principles.[1] It was only a matter of time before physical education would jump onto the Progressive bandwagon.

THE "NEW PHYSICAL EDUCATION"

Thomas Wood, Luther Halsey Gulick, and Clark Hetherington were among the leading progressive physical educators. They believed in natural activities (running, jumping, throwing, striking), which formed the basis of sports and athletic skills. They promoted sports and games over gymnastics because they believed sporting activities would be more stimulating and attractive to students and at the same time satisfy the progressive character-building and social-development goals—namely, teamwork, cooperation, discipline, and commitment. The incorporation of sports and games into the curriculum became known as the **"new physical education."**

Wood, influenced largely by Dewey and William Kilpartrick at Columbia, laid the groundwork for a sports- and games-based curriculum in his 1910 treatise titled the "New Physical Education," which appeared in the *Ninth Yearbook of the National Society for the Study of Education.* Wood's document established natural activities through the medium of sports and games as the basis of the physical education curriculum. Wood's protégé, Clark Hetherington, who also studied under Hall, enhanced the conception of a natural activities curriculum through his research, teachings, and writings. Known as the "modern philosopher of physical education," Hetherington constructed a philosophical schematic in which physical education was the fundamental principle of education upon which character development and intellectual skills were built.[2]

Even before Wood and Hetherington articulated their visions of a sports-based curriculum, Luther Halsey Gulick had already begun to implement such programs. As director of the Springfield YMCA Training School, he asked James Naismith to develop a new game to keep young men active during the winter months between football and baseball seasons.

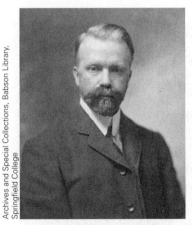

Archives and Special Collections, Babson Library, Springfield College

Luther Halsey Gulick

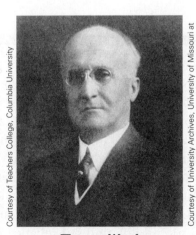

Courtesy of Teachers College, Columbia University

Thomas Wood

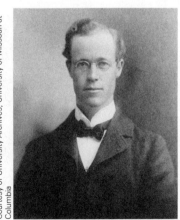

Courtesy of University Archives, University of Missouri at Columbia

Clark Hetherington

These three men promoted the new physical education with the injection of sports and games into the curriculum.

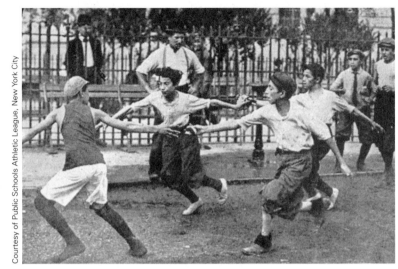

Courtesy of Public Schools Athletic League, New York City

The Public School Athletic League program in action.

In response Naismith created the game of basketball. Later in his career, Gulick, as the head of physical education for New York City schools, organized the Public Schools Athletic League (PSAL) in 1903 and incorporated natural activities into the classes. Two years later, he encouraged Elizabeth Burchanel to establish the girls' branch of PSAL. At its height, the PSAL served 600,000 students in the city's 630 schools. Its structure served as a prototype that seventeen other cities adopted.[3]

SOCIAL BENEFITS OF ATHLETICS

The PSAL embodied the social goals of Progressivism. In an attempt to rescue youth—young males, in particular—mired in the squalor and crime of overcrowded and unsavory urban tenement districts, civic leaders, social workers, and educators organized programs that provided structure for adolescents during their free time. They believed extracurricular activities, particularly athletics, would not only instill order and direction in their daily routines but would also strengthen their character with discipline, responsibility, and self-reliance. In New York City, Gulick used school athletics to channel youth from troublesome gangs into constructive endeavors.[4]

What Gulick offered the youth of New York City, Edwin Bancroft Henderson brought to African American children in Washington, D.C. A progressive with views similar to Gulick's, Henderson instituted physical education programs and athletic competitions to mold character, enhance citizenship, nurture social skills, and facilitate learning. Familiar with Gulick's athletic league prototype, he established a PSAL in Washington in 1910.[5] Henderson's action reflected the spread of interschool athletics across the United States, a movement that forced school administrators to rationalize the existence of interscholastic athletic programs with a doctrine that packaged athletics in educational wrappings.

THE "ATHLETICS ARE EDUCATIONAL" DOCTRINE

The **"athletics are educational" doctrine** not only enabled educators to defend the existence of athletic programs, but also gave them ample ammunition to call for their expansion. From 1906 to 1939, athletic programs in high schools increased markedly, due chiefly to the United States' shift in attitude toward ruggedness, nature, and virility, embodied in Theodore Roosevelt's call for the "strenuous life"; the work of the Playground Association of America founded by Gulick in 1906 (later National Recreation Association) in promoting sport and public recreation as an antidote to some of society's problems; the expansion of athletic programs at YMCAs; and the adoption of physical education curricula with emphasis on sports and games rather than gymnastics. During the nineteenth century, physical education emerged in the public school systems independently of athletics, but in the twentieth, it dovetailed naturally with athletics to form a logical union.[6]

In actuality, though, the advent of athletics stimulated the growth of physical education—a growth that school administrators welcomed and encouraged, for they saw physical education as a useful medium for regulating athletics. Administrators began to hire athletic coaches as full-time physical education teachers, and such hirings enabled school officials to control a troublesome area. At the same time, the sports and games curriculum, with its capacity to accommodate large numbers of students in physical education classes, met the demands of increasing school enrollments.

Educators were forced to justify the existence of athletics, this new component in their schools. With athletic coaches on their faculties and sports and games in their curricula, they attached educational attributes to athletics, giving rise to the "athletics are educational" doctrine. For more than three generations, educators promulgated this doctrine, and athletics in no small way contributed to the expansion and visibility of physical education. Heightened visibility contributed, at least indirectly, to the adoption of state legislation that made physical education compulsory.

COMPULSORY PHYSICAL EDUCATION AND STATE LEGISLATION

By the time of World War I, a movement was already underway for compulsory physical education in the public schools. Some states enacted mandatory physical education laws in the nineteenth century—notably California (1866), Ohio (1892), Louisiana (1894), Wisconsin (1897), and North Dakota (1899). The movement for compulsory physical education laws gathered steam during the 1910s, when a combination of forces, nearly all related to military preparedness, pushed the issue to center stage. With wartime readiness the question of the day, government officials, military enthusiasts, and social critics believed that military training should be required in the public schools.

Early on, the American Physical Education Association (APEA), the forerunner of AAHPERD, promoted daily physical education over compulsory military training. It recommended "a rational system of physical training, consisting of exercises and games adapted to the age, sex, and a capacity of the growing boy and girl."[7] At its 1916 annual convention, APEA called upon states to enact required physical education laws. Later that year it appointed Dudley Sargent, James H. McCurdy, and APEA president William H. Burdick to a National Legislative Committee to examine and then make recommendations on all proposed national, state, and local legislation dealing with physical training. One year later, President Burdick criticized the profession for failing to inspire "a joy in physical training in the hearts of its pupils."[8]

But interest in state physical education legislation extended beyond the boundaries of APEA. Dudley Sargent, one of the Association's leading figures, along with John Dewey and six other prominent educators, organized the Committee for Promoting Physical Education in the Public Schools of the United States in response to President Woodrow Wilson's statement that "physical training is needed, but can be had without compulsory military service." Dewey chaired this august body, whose aim was to convince all state legislatures to require physical education without any military components.

The chief force in moving states to adopt mandatory physical education legislation, however, was the **National Physical Education Service.** It crystallized from a 1918 meeting of sixty national leaders who were invited to address the pleas of the U.S. Commissioner of Education for a nationwide interest in physical education and health. The Service, an arm of the Playground and Recreation Association (formerly Playground Association of America) and directed by James E. "Jimmy" Rogers, had a twofold mission. It promoted compulsory physical education laws on the state and federal levels, and it provided assistance to state departments of education for implementing statewide programs under the supervision of state directors of physical education. Rogers traveled throughout the United States, consulting state education departments and urging state legislators to adopt compulsory physical education laws.[9]

This movement for compulsory physical education reached a crescendo during World War I, when the medical examiner's report revealed that one-third of the inductees (1 of 3 million) were declared unfit for service. The poor showing on the induction examination, in combination with the efforts of APEA, the National Physical Education Service, and special-interest legislative committees led to increased state legislation. By 1930, thirty-six states had adopted compulsory physical education laws, enhancing the profession's credibility.[10]

EARLY SCIENTIFIC APPROACHES AND CREDIBILITY

As state legislation elevated physical education in the public sphere, professionals began to establish a link between scientific knowledge and physical education in order to obtain status and credibility for the existence of their discipline in the curriculum. Through testing and measuring psychomotor skills (throwing, catching, striking, kicking, and the like), strength, speed, and other physical attributes, professionals justified offering academic credit for physical education courses. Although anthropometric measurement and strength testing date back to nineteenth-century pioneers, the educational testing movement that was part of progressivism in education spilled into physical education after the First World War. During the 1920s, Sargent, dissatisfied with early strength tests, developed the Sargent jump to measure power and efficiency. Charles McCloy applied statistical methods to physical education in order to develop achievement scales. Frederick Rand Rogers, borrowing items from Sargent's strength test, developed his Physical Fitness Index (PFI) and used it to classify students for creating balance in competitive situations. Rogers used his PFI and D. K. Brace employed his battery of motor ability tests for homogeneous groupings. McCloy classified students on the basis of a weighted formula for age, weight, and height. Agnes Wayman devised a physical efficiency test for college women, and the National Recreation Association developed National Physical Achievement Standards for boys in a variety of physical activities.[11]

While measurement and evaluation brought some credibility and status to physical education, the profession, as a whole, did not develop a solid scientific foundation upon which to build its principles. Nonetheless, three individuals—Arthur Steinhaus at George Williams College (1923), Coleman Griffith at the University of Illinois (1925–32), and James H. McCurdy at Springfield College (1927) established research laboratories to investigate physical activity and sport. McCurdy and Steinhaus studied physical attributes, while Griffith's interest lay in the psychological. All three laboratories were short-lived, lasting from one to eight years, but they reveal that some physical educators turned to scientific inquiry in the early days of the profession.[12]

Operating concurrently with those early research laboratories was the **Harvard Fatigue Laboratory,** which opened in 1927. But unlike those first three, it was not associated with any physical education programs. The brainchild of Lawrence J. Henderson, M.D., director of the department of physical chemistry at the Harvard Medical School, the laboratory was established to study performance in the workplace. Under the leadership of D. B. Dill, the laboratory's research director, most of the early research focused on blood chemistry, work physiology, and fatigue. When World War II broke out, the laboratory channeled its research to the war effort. It investigated the effects of cold and altitude on clothing and equipment, analyzed foodstuffs and nutrition for sustenance, examined physical fitness limitations, and probed the transport of gases by the blood. The laboratory closed in 1947, when newly hired university administrators viewed the laboratory as no longer important to Harvard's mission.[13]

In its twenty years of existence, the Harvard Fatigue Laboratory laid the foundation for physiology of exercise. In 1931 Dill and Arlie Bock, professor at the medical school and director of the Medical Laboratory at Massachusetts General Hospital, revised F. A. Dainbridge's 1919 monograph, *The Physiology of Muscular Exercise,* perhaps the earliest text on exercise physiology. But one of the laboratory's greatest contributions was the apprenticeship opportunities it provided for a number of physiologists—such as Sid Robinson at Indiana University, H. L. Taylor at the University of Minnesota, and Steven Horvath at the University of California, Santa Barbara—who then established exercise physiology laboratories at institutions around the country. These offshoots played no small role in turning some physical educators toward the hard sciences. At the same time, however, physical education embraced the social and behavioral sciences.[14]

Social and behavioral goals, rooted in Progressivism, permeated education and impregnated the educational designs of Wood and Hetherington in forming the basis of the "new physical education." Following World War I, a new generation of scholars, led by Rosalind Cassidy, Jesse Feiring Williams, and Jay B. Nash, moved forward to carry the profession's torch. In 1927 Cassidy and Wood published their influential text, *The New Physical Education: A Program of Naturalized Activities toward Physical Education*. Williams, at Columbia University's Teachers College, kept alive Wood's thesis that physical education was a part of education with his own trademark shibboleth, "education *through* the physical." Nash, a protégé of Hetherington's, upheld the "new physical education," extending its tenets beyond the school day to evening and weekend recreation programs for youth. A strong believer in the principles of democracy, Nash looked upon the athletic field and gymnasium as great laboratories for fostering social intercourse and cultivating cooperation, character, and citizenship. On another front, he accepted the challenges presented by increased leisure time, moving into the vanguard of the profession and educating the American public on effectively using this time through publications and lectures. Just as newfound leisure time changed American life, the nature and scope of athletic competition changed markedly during the postwar years, finding an expanded role with far-reaching implications for American society.[15]

ATHLETICS AND THE GOLDEN ERA OF SPORT

The 1920s have often been dubbed sport's golden era. In recovering from the horrors of World War I, the United States cast aside Victorian values that had guided its moral standards throughout most of the nineteenth century and into the early decades of the twentieth. The country experienced a social revolution in manners and morals that saw drastic changes in women's dress, sexual mores, alcohol consumption, and tobacco use. These changes, in combination with the Red Scare, racial tensions triggered by the revival of the Ku Klux Klan, cyclical patterns of economic boom and bust, and the overt and defiant activities of organized crime, created an unsettling and unstable atmosphere for most Americans. In times of instability, the public often searches for popular heroes—public figures who inspire confidence or bring a perception of stability to offset feelings of uncertainty. Never was this more apparent than during the 1920s.

Though Americans turned to a figure like Charles Lindbergh to bring them a sense of stability and reassure them of their security, several other figures emerged from the sports world and served the same purpose. Babe Ruth in baseball, Jack Dempsey in boxing, and Red Grange in football were the most prominent. They all came from humble backgrounds, made it big, and became household names. They symbolized power, force, and mastery of their own destiny. They gave Americans hope for success and assuaged their anxieties during a turbulent era. On the feminine side of the ledger, Suzanne Lenglen, Helen Wills, and Gertrude Ederle, with their spectacular performances, exemplified freedom for women. In 1926 Ederle became the fifth person and first woman to swim the English Channel, and she did it in record time. Lenglen and Wills, tennis titans of the era, challenged traditional deportment with their aggressive play. In a slap at the old guard, Lenglen, wearing revolutionary tennis costumes, personified the flapper on the tennis court.[16]

Red Grange, Knute Rockne, and the Four Horseman primed the pumps of collegiate football as universities across the country erected stadiums to accommodate upwards of 60,000 spectators. The number of stadiums doubled and gate receipts tripled during the 1920s. Big-time athletic programs supported by big money, though, were vulnerable to nefarious practices. Commercial interests, which began to dominate collegiate athletics, ushered in elite players who cared little about scholarship, as well as high-salaried collegiate coaches whose raison d'être was winning. As commercialism infected athletic programs, abuses mounted. Pleas for reform intensified after the 1929 Carnegie Report on *American College Athletics* exposed the disproportionate share of revenue that athletic programs squandered on training tables, travel, and equipment, not to mention the time and energy that went into practices and game preparation. Precisely those negative features of men's collegiate athletics prompted female physical educators to emphasize participation rather than competition in programs for girls and women.

WOMEN'S ATHLETICS AND THE DEBATE OVER PARTICIPATION VERSUS COMPETITION

As far back as the late nineteenth century, female physical educators sought control of athletics for women. Not only did they seek to avoid abuses common to men's programs, but, influenced by the democratic principles of John Dewey's educational doctrine, they also adopted a "sports for all" approach in which each player got to play. In addition, medical opinion about rigorous activities damaging women's childbearing organs and the Victorian idea that it was improper for women to engage in "manly" sports pushed women's programs toward a noncompetitive model. By the 1920s, this model took the form of **play days** and later **sports days.**[17]

Play days were social functions in which female students from several colleges gathered to participate in sporting and social activities. Rather than representing their respective schools, students formed composite teams whose membership consisted of at least one representative from each institution. All the teams then played each other and the contests thus became exhibition matches in which participation was more important than victory. Afterward, the students socialized and exchanged pleasantries over refreshments.

Play days were an outgrowth of female physical educators' struggle to wrest control of women's athletics away from the men who coached and administered women's competitive teams in the Amateur Athletic Union (AAU) or community-based programs. The battle heightened after the 1922 Women's Olympics in Paris, which attracted 22,000 spectators. Female physical educators, notably Kathleen Sibley and Blanche Trilling, criticized the event for the immodest costumes that young women wore, while engaging in undignified, aggressive behavior in competitive athletic venues. But the success of the games not only escalated female physical educators' desire to control women's sports, it also encouraged male-controlled sports bodies—the International Olympic Committee (IOC) and the AAU—to step up their efforts to govern women's sports. The IOC scheduled five women's track and field events at the 1928 Games at Amsterdam, beginning with a modest number to avoid the perception of excess that shrouded women's sports at Paris. The AAU initiated women's track and field championships in 1924.[18]

Female physical educators waged a counteroffensive for control of women's athletics through two interlocking organizations within and outside of physical education. The **Committee on Women's Athletics (CWA)** was formed in 1917 within the American Physical Education Association. The Women's Division of the **National Amateur Athletic Federation (NAAF)** came into being in 1923, a year after the parent body was organized to challenge the AAU for control of amateur sport. Lou Henry Hoover served as titular head of the Women's Division, but Blanche Trilling, Ethel Perrin, Agnes Wayman, and four other female physical educators, all active in CWA, joined her on the Division's executive committee and inculcated their philosophy of noncompetitive athletics. Opposed to the commercialism and elitism of men's programs and fearing sexual exploitation that might occur with young females clad in skimpy outfits before the public's eye, they sought to protect girls and young women in the cloistered atmosphere of the play day. Subscribing to their motto, "Every Girl in a Sport and A Sport for Every Girl," they fulfilled their objective of providing noncompetitive or limited competitive athletic programs for women through play days and telegraphic meets; the latter enabled schools to conduct the activities at home and report the results—heights, distances, and times of track and field events, for instance—to participating schools via telegraph to determine the victor. In the 1930s and 40s, sports days replaced play days. In this venue, students represented their own school, but here, too, the primary objectives were socialization and participation.[19]

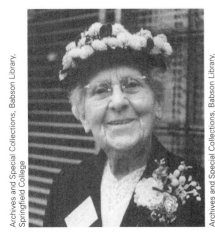

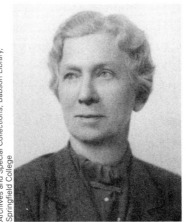

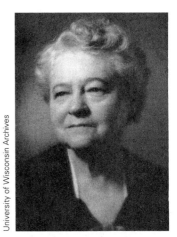

Ethel Perrin   Agnes Wayman   Blanche Trilling

These women guided women's athletics toward a participation rather than a competition model.

Mabel Lee, first female president of APEA, documented the anticompetitive sentiment among college women in two surveys she conducted in 1923 and 1931. Both showed overwhelming opposition to intercollegiate athletics, and the percentage of colleges participating in intercollegiate athletics declined by 10 percent over the eight-year period. Lee used these results to promote her philosophy of noncompetitive "educational," rather than "competitive," athletics.[20]

While white, middle-class colleges embraced play days and sports days, most black colleges followed the competitive model for their female athletes. African American female physical educators tended to work with their male colleagues in stressing competitive athletics as a proving ground for leadership positions in black communities. Moreover, through athletics, they could prepare prospective teachers to coach and administer interscholastic athletic programs in black elementary and high schools where limited resources made interscholastics the primary, if not the only, form of physical activity. Tuskegee Institute's program dominated competitive athletics for women prior to World War II.[21]

WORLD WAR II AND THE RENEWAL OF FITNESS

The advent of World War II brought about a renewed emphasis on fitness. Americans did poorly on the induction examination, and again nearly one-third of the inductees (nearly 3 out of 9 million) were deemed unfit for service. In 1940, after the outbreak of war in Europe, President Franklin D. Roosevelt appointed John B. Kelly, rowing medalist in the 1924 Olympics and father of Grace Kelly (who would become Princess Grace of Monaco), the National Director of Physical Training. But with no staff or resources, Kelly could do little. After Pearl Harbor Roosevelt put teeth into the fitness movement with a two-pronged government offensive. In 1942 he created the Division of Physical Fitness to generate nationwide interest in health and fitness through programs aimed at schools, colleges, and communities, and then in 1943 he called upon Kelly to head the Committee of Physical Fitness, which delivered information and services to schools and communities.[22]

Within the military itself, the government used professional physical educators to conduct physical training, sports, and recreation programs for the troops. C. H. McCloy, D. K. Brace, and others developed performance tests and served as fitness consultants for the armed forces. Women's branches of the armed services relied on the National Section of Women's Sports of the American Association of Health, Physical Education, and Recreation (AAHPER) for rules, standards, and policies regarding sports and recreation. Navy preflight V-12 training programs were housed at universities and colleges in which physical educators played important roles.[23]

The war effort, no doubt, enhanced physical education. Among the benefits accrued were increased time allotment for physical education, particularly in high schools; a greater percentage of students enrolled in physical education classes; and academic credit for physical education coursework. Professional preparation also improved: Standards were set for undergraduate teacher education programs in physical education, health education, and recreation. The proliferation of graduate programs, too, led the profession to develop standards and guidelines for graduate study in physical education.

As professional physical education reaped the benefits of war, America's interest in fitness began to wane, though not from within the profession. In 1943, AAHPER issued a statement at the National War Fitness Conference about the importance of physical fitness. Two years later AAHPER and the Educational Policy Commission issued a joint statement urging schools to require physical examinations and follow-ups, offer instruction in physical and mental health, and provide students with opportunities for play and exercise. In 1950 AAHPER and the Society of State Directors of HPER adopted a platform that reaffirmed the Association's fitness statements of 1943 and 1945. Unfortunately, AAHPER's message went unheeded.[24]

THE KRAUS-WEBER TESTS AND THE FITNESS EXPLOSION

The results of the **Kraus-Weber Test of Minimum Muscular Fitness** shocked the United States in 1953. In that year, Hans Kraus and Ruth Hirschland (also known as Bonnie Prudden) published their findings, which revealed a failure rate of 56.6 percent for American schoolchildren in comparison with 8.2 percent of their European counterparts. If a child failed one item on the six-item test, the child failed the test. American children, by and large, failed the standing toe-touch, while European children, groomed in gymnastics, had little difficulty in performing that task. Nevertheless, the results of the test ignited a fitness explosion.[25]

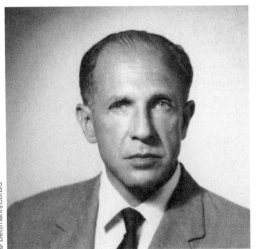
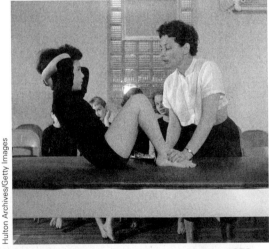

© Bettmann/Corbis

Hulton Archives/Getty Images

Hans Kraus and Bonnie Prudden sparked a fitness explosion during the 1950s, when they published the results of their fitness test.

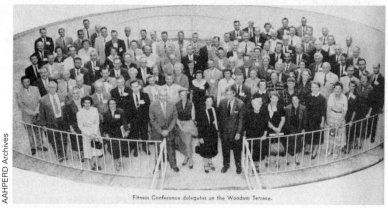

Fitness Conference delegates on the Woodner Terrace.

AAHPERD Archives

AAHPER Youth Fitness Conference

As news of the United States' miserable performance circulated across the country, John Kelly notified President Dwight D. Eisenhower, who summoned a group of athletes, sports writers, and sports authorities to a White House luncheon in July, 1955. Vice President Richard Nixon accepted the task of developing a national fitness program, and in September, 1956, the **President's Council on Youth Fitness** emerged from the President's Conference on Physical Fitness held at Annapolis.

Although AAHPER delegates attended the Annapolis conference and supported the fitness movement, the Association summoned more than a hundred of its own members to Washington. This body created the AAHPER Youth Fitness Project and later AAHPER's Operation Fitness program. Led by Paul Hunsicker, the Youth Fitness Project devised the AAHPER Youth Fitness Test, administered it to 8,500 children, and established norms. Coming to fruition in 1959, Operation Fitness combined camping and related outdoor activities with fitness testing. AAHPER distributed fitness testing kits, films, and other teaching aids, as well as promotional literature, to organizations interested in establishing and conducting fitness programs.[26]

At the state level, physical fitness also received great emphasis. California, Oregon, and New York developed fitness tests for pupils in their public schools. In New Haven, Connecticut, the public schools initiated a fitness program in which college students from nearby Southern Connecticut

State College helped schoolchildren improve their strength, endurance, and flexibility. But the classic fitness program was developed at LaSierra High School in Carmichael, California. Conceived by Stan LeProtti, physical education director and football coach, the LaSierra program rewarded boys with colored gym trunks for reaching designated fitness standards. Through this system of "group status," LeProtti contended, the average, nonathletic youngster with gold trunks, awarded for the highest fitness achievement, commands as much respect as the football hero. Designed to develop strength, endurance, power, agility, and balance with a minimum of 15 minutes of vigorous exercise daily, the LaSierra program spread to more than 200 schools across the country.[27]

FROM YOUTH FITNESS TO AEROBICS

Emphasis on youth fitness received an added boost from President John F. Kennedy in the early 1960s, when he deemed it vital for the defense of a nation mired in a cold-war struggle against communism. In his notable essay on fitness, "The Soft American" which appeared in *Sports Illustrated*, he castigated softness as a "menace to our security."[28]

The nature of fitness and exercise changed during the late 1960s. In 1968 Kenneth Cooper published **Aerobics,** the seminal work that translated physiological measurements of the body's ability to use oxygen into language the layperson could understand. Aerobic exercise—for instance, distance running—requires the body to take in oxygen and deliver it to the muscles in order for performance to continue. By converting measures of oxygen consumption, which physiologists use to gauge cardiovascular efficiency, into a simplified point system, Cooper made it possible for the average American to understand and determine how much cardiovascular endurance exercise was necessary in order to bring their heart, lungs, and blood vessels to efficient operating levels and thereby reduce, if not prevent, the onset of cardiovascular diseases. His thirty-point per week system consisted of performing any combination of walking, running, cycling, rowing, or other sporting activi-

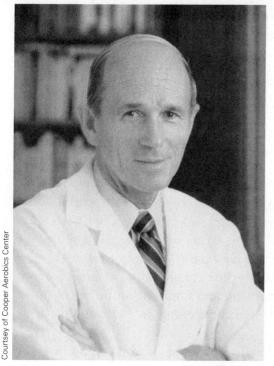

Courtesy of Cooper Aerobics Center

Only after you've measured exercise in terms of essential benefits to your body -- and that is what this book is all about -- will you understand why some of the most popular forms of exercise are almost worthless and why others, more neglected, score very high. Until now, not even the best exercise book -- not even your own physician -- could answer the question: "What form of exercise and how much will improve my health and protect my life?" Here, at last, is the answer.

Aerobics

a scientific program of exercise aimed at the overall fitness and health of your body with a unique point system for measuring your progress towards maximal health

Kenneth H. Cooper, M.D., M.P.H., Major, U.S. Air Force

Introduction by Richard L. Bohannon, SURGEON GENERAL U.S.A.F. (Ret.)

Preface by Senator William Proxmire

Courtesy of Cooper Aerobics Center

Ken Cooper and his book *Aerobics*, revolutionized exercise and training in the United States.

ties. With this user-friendly system, virtually anyone could participate and determine his or her own fitness level by performing a twelve-minute run periodically and comparing the distance covered with a time chart based on age and gender categories.[29]

Cooper's *Aerobics* revolutionized exercise practices in this country, and adults of all ages turned to jogging, cycling, swimming, and other aerobic activities. The surge in jogging led to the formation of running clubs, which, in turn, led to the popularity of marathons, initiated by the New York City marathon in 1971. The number of health spas proliferated, and Americans went through tennis and racquetball fads. But Cooper's work also changed the way in which physical educators taught fitness. They moved from the calisthenic (pull-up, push-up, sit-up) approach to cardiovascular endurance training programs, though strength, flexibility, and muscular endurance activities continue to be part of what today is considered health-related fitness. As the direction of fitness changed during the 1960s, so, too, did the nature of competitive athletics, especially for women.

THE FEMINIST MOVEMENT AND THE QUEST FOR EQUALITY IN ATHLETICS

Until the early 1960s, most girls' and women's athletic programs followed the participation model of the play day and sports day, though there were some early attempts to make women's sports competitive. In 1941 Gladys Palmer of Ohio State University proposed intercollegiate competition for women through the auspices of a Women's Collegiate Athletic Association. She also arranged a collegiate golf tournament to determine the national champion. In spite of opposition from female physical educators at large, Palmer held the golf tournament, and following a brief interruption during the war years, it resumed in 1946 and has been held annually.[30]

Though isolated and sporadic pockets of competitive athletics for women existed, the participation model remained in vogue. The 1964 Civil Rights Act and the feminist movement, the formation of the National Organization for Women (NOW), and the Equal Pay Act of 1963 moved the issue of gender equality in sport to center stage. Through the forum of equal rights, women began calling for funding, equipment, facilities, and resources comparable to those of men's sports programs. Even before the feminist movement hit full stride, a cadre of female physical educators, headed by Celeste Ulrich, Katherine Ley, Phoebe Scott, and Sara Jernigan, promoted varsity athletics for girls and women. Their advocacy led in 1966 to the formation of the **Commission for Intercollegiate Athletics for Women (CIAW),** a subunit of the Division of Girls and Women's Sports (DGWS) within AAHPER.[31]

During the late 1960s the National Collegiate Athletic Association (NCAA), in a long-standing feud with the Amateur Athletic Union for control of amateur athletics, hatched a plan to take complete control of amateur sport by inviting CIAW to affiliate with it. CIAW, under the leadership of Katherine Ley,

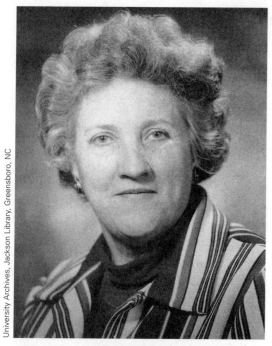

University Archives, Jackson Library, Greensboro, NC

Celeste Ulrich

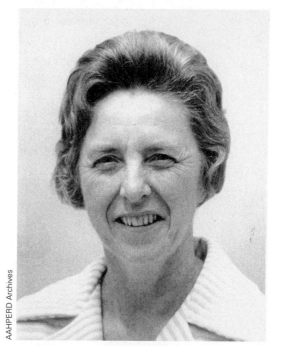

AAHPERD Archives

Katherine Ley

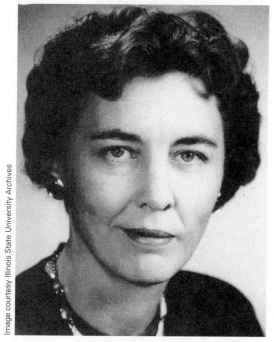

Image courtesy Illinois State University Archives

Phoebe Scott

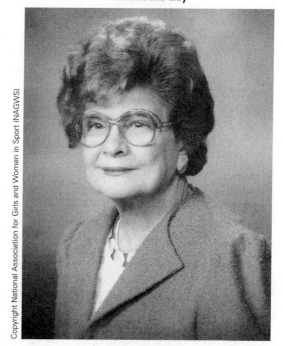

Copyright National Association for Girls and Women in Sport (NAGWS)

Sara Jernigan

Four women who led the movement toward competitive athletics for women.

viewed affiliation with NCAA as a mechanism for losing control of women's athletics. In a counter-move, CIAW decided to hold its own national championships. Then in an effort to bring more direction and stronger governance to women's sports, it reconstituted itself in 1971 into the **Association for Intercollegiate Athletics for Women (AIAW).** With Carole Oglesby as its first president, it continued to hold national championships, but it opposed athletic scholarships for women until 1973, when a female athlete's suit forced AIAW to accept scholarship athletes.[32]

In 1972 the federal government passed **Title IX of the Education Amendments Act,** which required institutions to provide equal opportunities and equal funding for all programs or activities receiving federal financial assistance. Educational institutions had until 1978 to bring their programs into compliance with Title IX. Although some collegiate programs moved toward compliance, most ignored the edict, as did the NCAA, until the early 1980s, when women's programs began to gather momentum. In 1980 the NCAA announced that it would hold national championships for small colleges (Division II and III), and the following year it decided to hold national championships for the major colleges (Division I). This move destroyed AIAW, which did not have the resources to compete with the larger and stronger NCAA, and it alienated female administrators and some coaches who saw their control of women's athletics co-opted by the male-dominated NCAA.[33]

Then, in 1984 the Supreme Court ruled in *Grove City v. Bell* that non-federally funded programs did not have to comply with Title IX, which prompted institutions to eliminate federal funding from their athletic programs. Four years later, however, Congress passed—over President Ronald Reagan's veto—the Civil Rights Restoration Act, placing athletics under the jurisdiction of Title IX. More recently, the **Equity in Athletics Disclosure Act of 1996** requires colleges and universities to show how they will meet the "substantial proportionality" test. This legislation calls for the proportion of female athletes to be within 5 percent of the institution's female enrollment. Nowhere has the im-

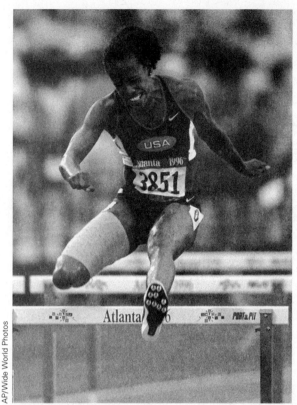

AP/Wide World Photos

Jackie Joyner Kersee, heptathlon victor and word's elite all-round athlete.

pact of Title IX been more visible than in the recent Olympic Games.[34]

A CENTURY OF OLYMPIC COMPETITION

Female athletes, reaping the benefits of Title IX, which saw numerous competitive sport opportunities proliferate for young girls during the 1970s and 1980s, demonstrated their tenacity at the Centennial Olympics in Atlanta, capturing gold medals in soccer, softball, and basketball. Over the years— from Babe Didrikson's triumphs in the 1932 games to Jackie Joyner Kersee's sparkling performances in the heptathlon in 1988 and 1992—women have left their mark on Olympic competition.

Even though superlative performances are intended outcomes of Olympic competition, the modern Games have been shrouded in nationalism and political machinations since their revival in 1896. Perhaps the gravest example of politicization came at Berlin in 1936 when Adolf Hitler attempted to use the Games as a showcase of Nazi propaganda. But in spite of Hitler's plan to demonstrate Aryan superiority through sport, Jesse Owens stole the spotlight, winning four gold medals and setting the world record in the long jump. Thirty-six years later, swimmer Mark Spitz won seven gold medals and set seven world records at the Munich games, where eleven Israeli athletes were slain at the hands of Arab terrorists. The games of the previous Olympiad at Mexico City in 1968 saw John Carlos and Tommie Smith protest the plight of African Americans back home with their black power salute on the victory stand. In the 1980s the United States and Soviet Union took turns boycotting each other's games in a demonstration of political one-upsmanship. The United States vowed it would not participate in the 1980 games in Moscow unless the Soviets withdrew its military

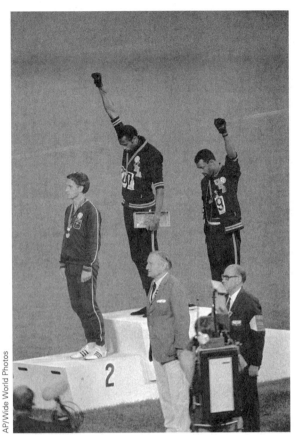

AP/Wide World Photos

Tommie Smith and John Carlos
in a Black Power salute at the
Mexico City Games, 1968.

forces from Afghanistan, which it had recently invaded. When the Soviets refused, the United States and sixty-one other nations, including Canada, West Germany, and Japan, stayed home. Four years later the Soviets retaliated by not sending a team to the Los Angeles Olympics that produced effervescent gymnast Mary Lou Retton and stellar hurdler Edwin Moses. Joan Benoit won the first-ever women's marathon, and Carl Lewis duplicated Jesse Owens's feat of winning four track and field gold medals.[35]

The 1988 games saw Florence Griffith Joyner, with her flamboyant uniforms, decorative fingernails, and stylish hairdos, win gold in the 100- and 200-meter races, while Carl Lewis took gold in the long jump and 100 meters, the latter coming when Canada's Ben Johnson tested positive for steroid use, forcing him to forfeit the medal to Lewis.[36] The participation of professional athletes eliminated the question of amateurism by 1992, as NBA players headed by Michael Jordan, Charles Barkley, Karl Malone, and Patrick Ewing easily demolished all comers in capturing the gold medal at Barcelona. In spite of spectacular performances by its athletes, the Olympic Games, perennially involved in controversies over political abuse, hypocrisy, and corruption, have been besieged by criticism since their reincarnation. In a similar vein, physical education, as a profession, has borne the brunt of severe criticism during the latter half of the twentieth century.

THE JOCK MENTALITY AND PUBLIC CRITICISM

In the years following World War II, physical education became a haven for scholarship athletes whose academic abilities were suspect or whose interest in or concern for academic achievement was minimal. By the 1960s, the profession found itself beset with a dumb-jock, animalistic, macho image. The stereotypical physical education jock was perhaps best personified by Dick Butkus, an all-American linebacker at the University of Illinois. In a 1964 feature article, Butkus told *Sports Illustrated*, "If I was smart enough to be a doctor, I'd be a doctor. I ain't, so I'm a football player. They got me in PE."[37]

This perception was reinforced during the early 1980s when three professors discovered that University of Nevada–Las Vegas athletes took 30 percent of their course work in physical education, even though few majored in that discipline. "Deprived of P.E. credits," they concluded, "most of the basketball and some of the football players would likely be ineligible to play or to remain enrolled as students."[38] More recently, Murray Sperber, critic of collegiate athletics, likened certain physical education courses to a hideaway curriculum that enables athletes to remain eligible for competition. In fairness to the discipline, he believes physical education is a legitimate course of study when the courses are conducted seriously, but he objects to physical education courses taught by coaches and their assistants, which he designated "an area of massive academic abuse."[39]

Those perceptions doubtless contributed to the jock mentality commonly associated with physical education. Even worse were the performances of barely literate athletes in postgame interviews on national television. Not all athletes fit into the dumb-jock mold, nor were all physical education majors dumb jocks. Athletes honored as Academic All-Americans and those selected as Rhodes Scholars have demonstrated that the term *scholar-athlete* is not an oxymoron. Nevertheless, the academic achievements of certain athletes, however grand, could not dispel the jock stereotype firmly ingrained in the public's mind through conventional wisdom.

The jock invasion was but one obstacle confronting physical education following World War II. No less harmful was the public criticism levied at the profession. Although education itself had become their favorite whipping boy, critics wasted little time in berating physical education, generally housed within schools or colleges of education. Severe denunciations appeared in Albert Lynd's *Quackery in the Public Schools* (1953) and Arthur Bestor's *Restoration of Learning* (1956). Lynd resorted to ridicule in condemning physical education graduate theses and courses involving coaching or teaching sports skills. Bestor, on a more sincere note, questioned the proliferation of such vocational courses (which he termed "pseudo-subjects") as physical education, home economics, pedagogy, and an assortment of others. He blamed it on the free elective system that emerged during the late nineteenth century. However his biggest complaint centered on the issue of vocational courses, leading to the creation of vocational departments whose members sought equal recognition with faculty in the liberal arts and sciences. The harshest indictment came in James B. Conant's *Education of American Teachers* (1963), which advised universities to cancel all graduate programs in physical education.[40]

Two years before the appearance of Conant's work, the California legislature enacted into law John Fischer's bill that defined academic subject matter areas as natural sciences, social sciences (other than education and methodology), humanities, mathematics, and fine arts. Conspicuously missing was physical education. In fact, during the bill's hearings, California newspapers chastised physical education on a daily basis. Editorials denounced physical educators/coaches who were teaching physics, math, or foreign languages and chastised the public school system for selecting one-third of all its administrators from the ranks of physical education. The Fischer Act questioned the legitimacy of physical education, and the jock mentality tarnished its image. Together, they both threatened the profession's existence. With their own survival at stake, physical educators moved to enhance their image by divorcing their programs from athletics and aligning them with prestigious disciplines in academia, most notably science.[41]

THE SCIENTIZATION OF PHYSICAL EDUCATION

The movement toward the **scientization of physical education** began to change the focus of physical education sometime between the late 1950s and early 1960s. Jan Rintala, in

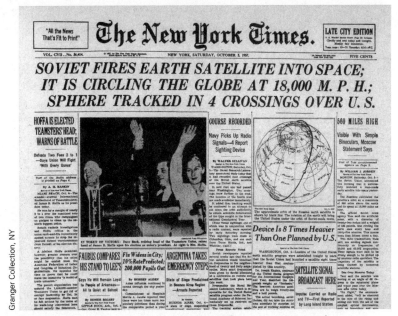

The launching of Sputnik shocked the United States into a science frenzy.

a *Quest* article, identified the beginning of this movement with the launching of *Sputnik* in 1957 and the enactment of the Fischer Bill in California in 1961. Roberta Park specified 1960 as the turning point, for in that year Warren Johnson published *Science and Medicine of Exercise and Sports,* and Raymond Weiss wrote "The Contributions of Physical Activity to Human Well-Being" for the *Research Quarterly Supplement.* Charles Corbin designated James B. Conant's 1959 Report on *The American High School* and Franklin Henry's oft-quoted piece, "Physical Education: An Academic Discipline," published in 1964 as indicators of the time when the profession began establishing its scientific basis.[42]

Changing demographics compelled college and university physical education programs to change their focus in order to stay in existence. As the demand for teachers decreased during the 1970s and 1980s, physical education turned toward the sciences to develop alternative professions and careers for its students in athletic training, sports management, corporate and adult fitness, and exercise gerontology. The multidisciplinary focus of those careers caused numerous physical education departments to change their names to exercise science or some variant of it in order to encompass the broader perspective their programs represented. With science-based physiology of exercise the core pillar of physical education, departments had to hire faculty with science backgrounds to teach courses in this area. Exercise physiologists, quite naturally, began looking to forums outside of AAHPERD to gather information and dispense their research. The most notable of these organizations was the American College of Sports Medicine (ACSM).

ACSM has its roots in physical education. Dudley Sargent, Edward Hitchcock, and Luther Gulick inspired R. Tait McKenzie, who in turn influenced ACSM founders Joseph Wolffe, Grover Mueller, and Arthur Steinhaus. Through the efforts of those individuals, ACSM evolved under the combined efforts of physical educators, physiologists, and cardiologists. Wolffe, a cardiologist at the Valley Forge Heart Institute and Hospital near Philadelphia, was most instrumental in bringing this organization to life. A member of the Federation Internationale Medico-Sportive et Scientifique (FIMS), he advanced a plan to form an American chapter of that association. Mueller, a physical education teacher in Philadelphia and ACSM's first executive secretary, assisted Wolffe in contacting physicians, physical educators, and physiologists who might have an interest in joining this organization. Steinhaus, a physiologist at George Williams College in Chicago, reinforced the idea of an American chapter of FIMS through his international travel and lectures. He soon developed a relationship with Swedish physician Ernst Jokl, who later emigrated to the United States. At the 1954 AAHPER Convention in New York, Jokl, Wolffe, Mueller, and Carl Troester, executive secretary of AAHPER, met to form an American chapter of FIMS. One year later, it became ACSM and since then has grown from eleven founders to more than 13,000 members.[43]

During the early decades of the century and long before the founding of ACSM, physicians with sports backgrounds offered their services to collegiate teams. At Harvard, Penn, Chicago, and several other universities, trainers, whose chief responsibilities involved conditioning and nutrition, joined "team doctors" in their efforts to treat and prevent athletes' injuries. Early books on athletic training began to appear during the 1910s, but athletic training did not begin to take on the character of a profession until the 1930s. In that decade definitive textbooks on the treatment and care of athletic injuries began to appear, and the Cramer Chemical Company of Gardner, Kansas, began publishing *The First Aider*—a newsletter that disseminated invaluable practical information for athletic trainers. In 1938 at the Drake Relays, athletic trainers from around the country organized themselves into the National Athletic Trainers Association (NATA), which functioned until World War II hastened its temporary demise in 1944. By the decade's end, however, trainers renewed their interest in the national association and resurrected NATA in 1950. Charles Cramer, the driving force behind the movement, became the organization's first national secretary. In 1959 the first educational program for athletic trainers was established.[44] Today, there are more than eighty-five curriculum programs scattered across the United States. In recent years the Commission for the Accreditation of Allied Health Education Programs (CAAHEP) has assumed the responsibilities of accrediting and reaccrediting athletic-training curriculum programs. NATA developed standards for athletic trainers and began certifying them in 1970.

Joining athletic training and sports medicine in the curriculum during the 1960s was sports management. Pioneered at Ohio University in 1966, sports administration and facilities management apply the business principles of organization, marketing, management, finance, and budgeting to sports and athletic programs.

Just as physical education's professional preparation has expanded to multidimensional career options, its academic face has become multifaceted. Physical educators, schooled in history, sociology, psychology, and philosophy, joined their colleagues in those respective disciplines to form their own organizations. Here, the sport historian, sport psychologist, and other disciplined-based physical educators found a forum for expressing their ideas and an audience responsive to their research. Although subdisciplines have satisfied the academic needs of a great number of physical educators, they have also divided the profession, siphoning off members and perhaps even reducing its overall effectiveness. Throughout the twentieth century, as interest in physical education ebbed and flowed, the profession demonstrated great resilience in making necessary adjustments to survive.

SURVIVAL AND IDENTITY IN A MARKET ECONOMY

Supply and demand have always driven physical education. Throughout its history, it has responded out of necessity to the dictates of society. Repeatedly, it has redefined its purpose to meet the demands of changing economic and social conditions and, in essence, followed what John Naisbitt so aptly described as the "Law of the Situation."[45] When it was in physical education's best interests to adopt athletics at the turn of the century, it did so; when it was beneficial to embrace fitness and measurement after the two world wars because draftees scored poorly on physical examinations, it did so. When it was imperative to develop allied careers in the 1970s, whether in athletic training, sports management, or exercise programming for adults and older adults, it moved in those directions. Granted, some movement toward allied careers was voluntary, but most was driven by the drought of teaching positions that placed physical education in jeopardy. Its professionals had no alternative: Either adapt to societal changes and changes in the marketplace, or risk joining the ranks of the unemployed.

In the twenty-first century, the forces of a market economy will continue to prevail. In order to survive, physical education will need to promote itself in a world that has become increasingly competitive in both the public and private sectors. Mike Ellis, prominent physical educator and former dean at the University of Oregon, has urged the profession to reconceptualize itself as a "retail service." Due to changing demographic and lifestyle patterns in the United States, physical education "will have to follow the dictates of the market and . . . identify potential clients and turn them into regular customers."[46]

The emergence of the concept of **wellness** during the last quarter of the twentieth century and its growing emphasis in the twenty-first, expand the market of potential clients for physical education. Although wellness is a multidimensional concept involving intellectual, emotional, social, and spiritual components along with its physical attributes, physical educators must use their knowledge and abilities to stimulate physical activity in likely clients, converting them into customers who exercise on a regular basis. Moreover, the findings of the *Surgeon General's Report on Physical Activity and Health* (1996), combined with the objectives of *Healthy People 2000* (1990) and *Healthy People 2010* (2000), reinforce the notion that there is a ready-made market to tap. The two *Healthy People* reports call for increased physical activity and more healthy days per month for all age groups, while the Surgeon General's report reveals the necessity of physical activity. Even moderate amounts of daily physical activity can improve health and enhance the quality of life. Given that 60 percent of American adults do not engage in any leisure-time physical activity and less than 23 percent participate in a program of regular vigorous physical activity, and because fewer than 30 percent of American high school youth, grades 9–12, have daily physical education, the challenge lying before physical education is formidable.[47] Nevertheless, physical education has a golden opportunity to strengthen our nation's physical fabric through effective, stimulating, and accommodating exercise and physical activity programs that serve everyone. With its knowledge base and leadership, physical education has the capacity to devise, disseminate, and deliver physical activity programs that will enable Americans to preserve their health and enjoy wellness deep into the twenty-first century.

On the Web

www.aahperd.org
Site of American Alliance for Health, Physical Education, Recreation and Dance. Contains information on the profession of physical education, convention programs, and recent news items.

www.fitness.gov
Site of the President's Council on Physical Fitness and Sports. Contains information, news items, and discussion of research issues dealing with physical fitness and sporting activities.

http://www.health.gov/healthypeople/Publications
Contains the goals and objectives of Healthy People 2010.

www.sportshalls.com
Search engine to find sports museums and halls of fame.

Key Terms

Aerobics Kenneth Cooper's seminal work (1968) that popularized cardiorespiratory fitness in America by simplifying technical physiological measurements of the body's ability to use oxygen into easily understood concepts (page 106).

Association for Intercollegiate Athletics for Women (AIAW) An organization formed from CIAW in 1971 to bring more direction and governance to women's sports (page 110).

"athletics are educational" doctrine Belief that athletics had redeeming educational values; enabled school administrators and educators to justify the existence of interscholastic athletics (page 93).

Commission for Intercollegiate Athletics for Women (CIAW) A subunit of the Division of Girls and Women's Sports (DGWS) within AAHPER that was organized in 1966 to promote varsity athletics for girls and women (page 108).

Committee on Women's Athletics (CWA) A committee within the American Physical Education Association (APEA) organized in 1917 by female physical educators to maintain control of women's athletics (page 101).

Equity in Athletics Disclosure Act of 1996 Federal legislation that requires colleges and universities to meet the proportionality test in which the proportion of athletes in the underrepresented gender must be within 5 percent of the underrepresented gender's enrollment (page 110).

Harvard Fatigue Laboratory Physiology laboratory established at Harvard in 1927 to assess performance in the workplace; during World War II it turned to investigating the limitations of physical fitness, the effects of cold and altitude on clothing and equipment, and transport of gases in the blood. It closed in 1947, but its major contribution was to provide a training ground for physiologists who would establish the field of physiology of exercise (page 97).

Kraus-Weber Test of Minimum Muscular Fitness Tests administered to American and European schoolchildren in 1953 in which 56.6 percent of the Americans and 8.2 percent of the Europeans failed. Results of this test sparked a physical fitness explosion during the 1950s (page 104).

National Amateur Athletic Federation (NAAF) An organization founded in 1923 to challenge the Amateur Athletic Union (AAU) for control of amateur sport in America (page 101).

National Physical Education Service Supported by the Playground and Recreation Association and headed by James E. "Jimmy" Rogers, this organization emerged in 1918 to promote compulsory physical education and to assist state departments of education in the implementation of physical education programs (page 95).

new physical education Curriculum based on natural activities and sports and games that came into being during the Progressive era (page 91).

play days Social functions in which female students from several colleges gathered for sporting and social activities. They formed composite sports teams consisting of one player from each school and played exhibition matches against one another. Afterward, the students socialized over refreshments (page 100).

President's Council on Youth Fitness Organized in 1956 as one reaction to the performance of American schoolchildren on the Kraus-Weber test. Today, the agency is known at the President's Council on Physical Fitness and Sports (PCPFS) (page 105).

progressive education Movement that grew out of Progressivism and led by John Dewey, G. Stanley Hall, and others; it established a child-centered curriculum based on pupils' maturation levels to facilitate learning and prepare youth to function effectively in a democratic society (page 90).

Progressivism Reform movement of the late nineteenth and early twentieth century that produced significant changes in government, agriculture, banking, business, social services, urban housing, and education (page 90).

scientization of physical education The movement of physical education toward a scientific basis with the adoption of more science-oriented courses in the curriculum, affiliation with science-based professional organizations, and modification of departments' names to include science or some variation of it (page 114).

sports days Social functions that evolved from play days in which all female participants represented their respective schools, but participation rather than competition was emphasized (page 100).

Title IX of the Education Amendments Act of 1972 Federal legislation that mandated equal opportunities and equal funding for all programs or activities receiving federal financial assistance (page 110).

wellness Optimal health and total well-being, generally involving physical, intellectual, social, emotional, and spiritual dimensions (page 118).

Multiple Choice Questions

1. The "new physical education" emphasized
   a. sports and games
   b. formal gymnastics

    c. military drill

    d. b and c of the above

    e. a, b, and c of the above

2. The leaders of the "new physical education" were

    a. Luther Gulick

    b. Clark Hetherington

    c. Thomas Wood

    d. a and b of the above

    e. a, b, and c of the above

3. The African American progressive physical educator who instituted athletic competition in the Washington, D.C., schools was

    a. Paul Robeson

    b. Jackie Robinson

    c. Booker T. Washington

    d. W. E. B. DuBois

    e. Edwin Bancroft Henderson

4. The organization(s) that called for compulsory physical education in the schools before the 1917 Medical Examiner's Report was (were)

    a. National Physical Education Service

    b. APEA (forerunner of AAHPERD)

    c. Committee for Promoting Physical Education in Public Schools

    d. a and c of the above

    e. a, b, and c of the above

5. The Women's Division of the National Amateur Athletic Federation advocated

    a. competitive athletics

    b. international competition

    c. play days

    d. national championships

    e. poetry reading

6. The results of the Kraus-Weber test caused a reaction that led President Eisenhower to create the

    a. AAHPERD

    b. ACSM

    c. President's Council for Physical Fitness & Sports

    d. NCAA

    e. NATA

7. The organization for women's collegiate athletics that began sponsoring national championships in 1971 was

    a. AIAW

    b. NCAA

    c. NOW

    d. AAU

    e. GAR

8. The national legislation adopted in 1972 that called for equal funding of men's and women's collegiate athletic programs, if the institution received federal funds, was

    a. Title VI

    b. Title VII

    c. Title IX

    d. Y. A. Tittle

    e. Titletown

9. During the 1960s, the focus on physical fitness changed from calisthenic-type activities to

    a. aerobic activities

    b. anaerobic activities

    c. team sports

    d. weight training

    e. dance

10. In order for physical education to survive throughout the twenty-first century, the profession must find potential clients and turn them into

    a. successful athletes

    b. Rhodes scholars

    c. regular customers

    d. convincing hucksters

    e. capable administrators

Critical Thinking Questions

1. The "new physical education" grew out of the Progressive movement and Progressive education. Why did new physical education leaders, Thomas Wood, Clark Hetherington, and Luther Gulick move physical education toward a curriculum emphasizing natural activities and sports and games?

2. Why did female physical educators during the 1920s and 30s adopt participation models of "play days" and "sports days" for college women rather than the competitive model of intercollegiate athletics, and why were these models unacceptable by the 1960s?

3. The Kraus-Weber test spawned a physical fitness revolution in the 1950s, and Cooper's *Aerobics* in the late 1960s and 1970s triggered a movement toward cardiovascular fitness, yet less than 23 percent of American adults engage in regular, vigorous physical activity. Why do so many American adults refrain from regular, vigorous physical activity?

4. The profession of physical education has attempted to embrace the sciences in curriculum modification, affiliation with scientifically oriented professional organizations, and alteration of department names to show a connection to the sciences. Why has physical education gravitated toward the sciences?

5. Ever since its emergence as a profession, physical education has more or less followed the dictates of American society. Why has physical education been driven by the economic and social forces of our market economy, and what actions must the profession take in order to survive in the twenty-first century?

Notes and References

1. Arthur Weston, *The Making of American Physical Education* (New York: Appleton-Century-Crofts, 1962), 49–51.

2. Ibid., 51, 154–59.

3. J. Thomas Jable, "The Public Schools Athletic League of New York City: Organized Athletics for City Schoolchildren, 1903–1914," in *The American Sporting Experience: A Historical Anthology of Sport in America,* ed. Steven A. Riess (West Point, N.Y.: Leisure Press, 1984), 217–38.

4. J. Thomas Jable, "High School Athletics: History Justifies Extracurricular Status," *JOPERD,* 57, no. 2 (February 1986): 61–68.

5. David K. Wiggins, "Edwin Bancroft Henderson: Physical Educator, Civil Rights Activist, and Chronicler of African American Athletes," *Research Quarterly for Exercise and Sport,* 70, no. 2 (June 1999): 94–97.

6. Guy M. Lewis, "Adoption of the Sports Program, 1906–39: The Role of Accommodation in the Transformation of Physical Education," *Quest,* 12, no. 1 (May 1969): 34–46.

7. "Military Drill in Public Schools," *American Physical Education Review,* 21 (October 1916): 430.

8. William H. Burdick, "Editorial," *American Physical Education Review,* 22 (November 1917): 500.

9. J. Thomas Jable, "The AAHPERD: Professionals Proudly Promoting Physical Education," *The Physical Educator,* 38, no. 4 (December 1981): 205–06.

10. Deobold B. Van Dalen and Bruce L. Bennett, *A World History of Physical Education,* 2d ed. (Englewood Cliffs, N.J.: Prentice-Hall, 1972), 441.

11. Ibid., 468–71.

12. Walter P. Kroll, *Perspectives in Physical Education,* (New York: Academic Press 1971), 169–85.

13. Steven M. Horvath and Elizabeth C. Horvath, *The Harvard Fatigue Laboratory: Its History and Contributions* (Englewood Cliffs, N.J.: Prentice-Hall, 1973), 6–24, 77–84.

14. Ibid.

15. Van Dalen and Bennett, *World History of Physical Education*, 430–32; J. Thomas Jable, "Jay B. Nash," *JOPERD*, 56, no. 7 (September 1985): 55–57.

16. Benjamin G. Rader, *American Sports: From the Age of Folk Games to the Age of Spectators* (Englewood Cliffs, N.J.: Prentice-Hall, 1983), 176–93, 219–24, 237.

17. Ellen Gerber, "The Controlled Development of Collegiate Sport for Women, 1923–1936," *Journal of Sport History*, 2, no. 1 (Spring 1975): 1–28.

18. Mary H. Leigh and Therese M. Bonin, "The Pioneering Role of Madame Alice Milliat and the FSFI in Establishing Track and Field Competition for Women," *Journal of Sport History*, 4, no.1 (Spring 1977): 72–83; J. Thomas Jable, "Eleanor Egg: Paterson's Track and Field Heroine," *New Jersey History*, 102, nos. 3–4 (Fall-Winter 1984): 69–84.

19. Susan K. Cahn, *Coming on Strong: Gender and Sexuality in Twentieth-Century Women's Sport* (New York: Free Press, 1994), 55–68.

20. John A. Lucas and Ronald A. Smith, *Saga of American Sport* (Philadelphia: Lea & Febiger, 1978), 360.

21. Cindy Himes Gissendanner, "African-American Women and Competitive Sport, 1920–1960," in *Women, Sport, and Culture*, ed. Susan Birrell and Cheryl L. Cole (Champaign, Ill.: Human Kinetics, 1994), 81–92.

22. Jable, "The AAHPERD," 207.

23. Van Dalen and Bennett, 494, 507–08.

24. Jable, "The AAHPERD," 207.

25. Hans Kraus and Ruth Hirschland, "Muscular Fitness and Health," *JOPERD*, 24, no. 10 (December 1953): 17–19.

26. Jable, "The AAHPERD," 208.

27. Stanley Gordon, "La Sierra High Shows How Americans Can Get Physically Tough," *Look* (January 30, 1962): 49–62; Dorothy Barclay, "A City's Schools Get in Trim," *New York Times Magazine* (May 6, 1962).

28. John F. Kennedy, "The Soft American," *Sports Illustrated*, 13 (26 December 1960): 13–23.

29. Cooper, Kenneth H. *Aerobics* (New York: Bantam Books, 1968).

30. Lucas and Smith, 361–63.

31. Joan S. Hult, "NAGWS and AIAW: The Strange and Wondrous Journey to the Athletic Summit, 1950–1990," *JOPERD*, 70, no. 4 (April 1999): 25–26.

32. Ibid., 27–28; Ying Wu, "Early Attempts to Create a Women's Governance Plan, 1967—1973," *Proceedings of the North American Society for Sport History* (1997): 99–100.

33. Hult, 29–30.

34. Ibid.; *The Chronicle of Higher Education*, April 11, 1997.

35. Allen Guttmann, *The Olympics: A History of the Modern Games* (Urbana, Ill.: University of Illinois Press, 1992), 126–63.

36. Ibid., 165–74.

37. Dan Jenkins, "A Special Kind of Brute with a Love for Violence," *Sports Illustrated*, 12 October 1964, 32.

38. Joseph Raney, Terry Knapp, and Mark Small, "Pass One for the Gipper: Student-Athletes and University Course Work," in *Fractured Focus: Sport as a Reflection of Society*, ed. Richard Lapchick (Lexington, Mass.: Heath, 1986), 59.

39. Murray Sperber, *College Sports, Inc.: The Athletic Department vs. The University* (New York: Henry Holt, 1990), 283.

40. J. Thomas Jable, "Whatever Happened to Physical Education?" *Journal of Interdisciplinary Research in Physical Education*, 2, no. 1 (1997): 24.

41. Ibid.

42. Jan Rintala, "The Mind-Body Revisited," *Quest*, 43, no. 3 (December 1991): 268; Roberta J. Park, "On Tilting at Windmills While Facing Armageddon," *Quest*, 43, no. 3 (December 1991): 253; Charles B. Corbin, "The Field of Physical Education: Common Goals, No Common Roles," *JOPERD*, 42, no. 1 (January 1993): 84.

43. Jack W. Berryman, *Out of Many, One: A History of the American College of Sports Medicine* (Champaign, Ill.: Human Kinetics, 1995), 3–18.

44. Ibid., 30–31.

45. John Naisbitt, *Megatrends* (New York: Warner Books, 1982), 87–89.

46. Michael J. Ellis, "The Business of Physical Education," in *Trends toward the Future in Physical Education*, ed. John D. Massengale (Champaign, Ill.: Human Kinetics, 1987), 84.

47. U. S. Department of Health and Human Services, *Physical Activity and Health: A Report of the Surgeon General* (Atlanta: Centers for Disease Control and Prevention, National Center for Chronic Disease Prevention and Health Promotion, 1996); *Healthy People 2010*, http://www.health.gov/healthypeople

6

PHILOSOPHY AND ETHICS IN PHYSICAL EDUCATION

Chapter Objectives

After reading this chapter, the student will be able to

- Discuss what a philosophy is and why it is important
- Define four traditional philosophies
- Identify four branches of philosophy
- Explain what a personal philosophy is
- Begin the process of constructing and writing a personal philosophy
- Analyze a variety of ethical issues and related behaviors and determine appropriate behaviors
- Describe good and bad ethical traits

*P*hilosophy is one of the most basic, yet complex, terms in the English language. Everyone seems to know what **philosophy** is, but few really understand its actual meaning. For instance, nearly every adult and most teens can articulate what they believe to be their philosophy of life—more or less a moral code inculcated by their religious beliefs, parental influences, social customs, or local and national legislation. It generally contains principles about good and evil, right and wrong, acceptable and unacceptable behavior, the meaning of life and the best way to live life. In addition to these aspects of one's philosophy of life, the term *philosophy* has a much broader scope. For some, it is a position or viewpoint on a topic or an issue (such as capital punishment and abortion); for others it is a common element that identifies one with a particular cause (the environment, animal rights, or gun control); still others embrace it within the ideological framework of a political party or religious movement.

In the realm of physical education and sport, teachers and coaches banter about their philosophies on a routine basis. They frequently discuss their philosophical approaches to teaching fitness, movement, and/or motor-skill development in their physical education classes.

THE DISCIPLINE: PHILOSOPHICAL ANALYSIS

Philosophy, in its strictest sense, is the search for the truth; and we begin the search by following the four branches of the study (or discipline) of philosophy—metaphysics, epistemology, axiology, and logic. **Metaphysics** deals with the nature of reality—it asks questions about the relationship of mind and body, the existence of God, the possibility of personal immortality, the nature of being, even the origins of the universe. The traditional philosophies we will discuss all seek to answer metaphysical questions. The metaphysician searches for a way to determine what is real (is it the mind and ideas that are real, or is it the body and the physical world—or is it both?), and the philosophies that derive from these metaphysical questions help us decide what we accept as fact and as reality. **Epistemology** is the quest for

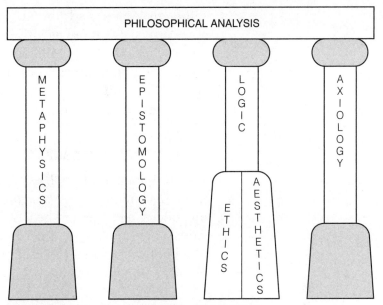

PHILOSOPHICAL ANALYSIS

METAPHYSICS

EPISTOMOLOGY

LOGIC

ETHICS

AESTHETICS

AXIOLOGY

Figure 6.1 Branches of the study of philosophy.

knowledge. It assists us in ascertaining the origin, nature, and structure of knowledge and verifying its validity. It asks questions about the difference between belief and knowledge, about the role of the senses in gaining knowledge, as well as the role of reason. Epistemology is closely related to metaphysics; the way we know the world must depend on the nature of the world. As a result, the traditional philosophies also have epistemological aspects. **Logic,** closely related to epistemology, is the study of thought processes and reasoning power and the process by which humans reach correct conclusions. Methods of reasoning are usually divided into deductive (a process whereby valid premises must lead to valid conclusions) and inductive reasoning (a process whereby the conclusion can be guaranteed only to a high degree of certainty). **Axiology** is the study of values, and it has several dimensions, two of which are ethics and aesthetics. **Ethics** deals with moral issues (questions of how we treat each other, the universality of moral values), while **aesthetics** is the study of the nature of art and beauty (questions of the role of art, the true meaning of an artwork, the beauty in an athletic performance).

Although "ethics" and "morals" are often used interchangeably, "ethics" is a more inclusive term. All four of these branches of the study of philosophy work together in the traditional philosophies (ways of viewing the world)—idealism, realism, pragmatism, existentialism, and humanism—as they search for truth.

TRADITIONAL PHILOSOPHIES

The traditional philosophies of idealism, realism, pragmatism, existentialism, and humanism provide a foundation for conceiving ideas and beliefs that ultimately allow individuals to formulate their personal philosophy; at other times in history, other philosophies have dominated the human search for truth.

Idealism

Idealism had its roots in ancient Greece, home of Socrates, Plato, and Aristotle; in the modern world, René Descartes, George Berkeley, Immanuel Kant, and Georg Hegel have been its leading representatives. Plato and other early idealists believed that ideas were the source of truth because earthly creatures and material items were imperfect. But in the mind, ideas could be cultivated, leading toward perfection. As the influences of the Judeo-Christian concept of God grew and spread in later centuries, idealism identified with the perfection and goodness of God. Therefore, the ideal represents that which is absolutely good. Human beings are real; they have a soul in addition to a mind and body, but the soul is actually an expression of the body. The idealist subscribes to a moral code or imperative that encourages good and shuns evil. Moral and spiritual values are important, and so is individual activity, which contributes to the development of the total self. Society serves as the medium for development, but it is also the beneficiary of one's self-improvement.

From an idealist approach, physical educators espouse and teach sportspersonship, fair play, and obedience to rules. Fitness and sports skills, though important, are not ends in themselves, but rather the means to spiritual and mental improvement. Idealist physical educators assume the central role in the learning process. They provide direction and guidance because they have the necessary knowledge and proper information that needs to be imparted. They rely largely on explanation and demonstration for teaching physical skills. In the classroom, lecture and assigned readings are the primary methodologies, but the physical educator also uses question-answer and class-discussion techniques as mechanisms for pursuing truth.

Realism

Realism is a reaction to idealism dating back to Aristotle; it holds that things exist in and of themselves, independent of the human mind. Other prominent realists were Thomas Aquinas, Michel de Montaigne, John Locke, Jean-Jacques Rousseau, and Herbert Spencer. Realists see knowledge in established facts. They have tangible goals; they are interested in measurement, evaluation, and statistics; they believe in tested methodologies and systematic teaching.

Physical educators who consider themselves realists stress physical fitness and motor-skill development from an early age. They believe in providing pupils with a wide range of physical activities. They encourage performance-based activities and learning through the use of all the senses. They believe anatomy, physics, biomechanics, statistics, and laboratory experiences are important for the preparation of physical education teachers because the sciences and measurement are crucial for providing experiences and evaluating progress. Realist physical educators promote values associated with the body and human movement. They stress wellness as an essential goal, with vigorous physical activity (cardiovascular endurance, strength, muscular endurance) serving as pathways to the fitness component of wellness. Relying upon science, the realists devise lessons and experiences that are objective and factual. They frequently assign student projects because they are definitive, measurable, and concrete. They also use films, videotapes, computer-generated programs, and other audio-visuals to reinforce or supplement their teaching. For the realist, the subject matter occupies the central position.

Pragmatism

The term *pragmatism* is derived from Greek words meaning "practice," or "practical." Emerging in the late nineteenth century, **pragmatism** is basically an American philosophy, emanating from the ideas of Charles Peirce, William James, and John Dewey. It holds that experience is the only source of truth, the only reality. All learning occurs through experience, the ultimate reality, and the more experiences one has, the better. The search for truth is a search for practical knowledge—for what will allow the individual to live a better life. Known also as experimentalism, pragmatism uses trial and error and problem solving to arrive at solutions that will help people achieve their goals.

A pragmatist changes as society changes, so values and morals may change as well. Because human beings are social animals, the social dimension of human nature needs cultivation for the betterment of society. Education occurs in a social setting and focuses on the child rather than subject matter. The school, then, has a primary role in preparing the learner to function effectively in a democracy, such as the United States, and to contribute constructively to society. The pragmatist physical educator provides certain essential experiences through physical activity that are not attainable in any other discipline. In addition to pursuing these unique goals, physical educators must also reach out to others in the educative process to establish communication channels and social relationships for interactive learning. Thus, group activities and team sports are highly desirable in a pragmatic curriculum, but individual, isolated activities, such as weight training, solitary distance running, or swimming laps, can also be incorporated with the establishment of effective socializing experiences. The pragmatist's selection of physical activities is far less important than the challenges, initiatives, and dilemmas that these experiences provide.

Existentialism

Existentialism focuses on how one finds meaning in an absurd world and on knowing the inner self. It grew from the work of Søren Kierkegaard, Friedrich Nietzsche, Martin

Heidegger, Jean-Paul Sartre, Franz Kafka, and Albert Camus. The existentialist sees life as frustrating, futile, and full of injustices that the individual cannot change or resolve. But the existentialist understands that one defines oneself through one's actions; the individual has the freedom of choice to accept responsibility for his or her own life and defines that life through what he or she does or chooses not to do. The existentialists seek self-realization in striving to always do the best they can.

For the existentialist in physical education, the individual self is the chief point of reference. One sets one's own standards in searching for creativity and free expression in physical activity and sports. For existentialists, dance, movement education, and play activities are best suited for free expression because the emphasis is on process rather than product or outcome. For some existentialists, competitive team games are less valuable because directing one's effort toward the team concept of winning deprives one of self-expression. But the existentialist might turn to competitive sports that afford self-selection of values and self-evaluation.

Humanism

Renaissance thought created an appreciation for human nature and a renewed respect for the human body through **humanism.** Although spiritual attributes continued to remain important, the image and stigma of a reprehensible human body, inculcated by the religious fervor of the Middle Ages, gradually dissipated, and scholars and artists emphasized human values. Today, in education, humanism is associated with an "open curriculum" and humanistic psychology, based on Abraham Maslow's tenets of self-actualization or striving for perfection of self. In physical education, human movement experiences promote self-actualization of the individual, and humanistic teachers seek to be compassionate and kind in addition to being knowledgeable about their discipline.

Other Traditional Philosophies

Other philosophies—naturalism, asceticism, and Scholasticism—have dominated thought during various periods of

Western civilization. **Naturalism,** the oldest philosophy, holds that all truth and reality are found in the laws of nature and in material things. Nothing exists beyond the physical universe; naturalism denies the concept of spirituality and the soul in human nature. In the modern period naturalism has evolved into realism and pragmatism. In the West, **asceticism** emerged with the rise of Christianity and the monastic movement and reached its peak during the Middle Ages. It emphasized spiritual development and the suppression of animal instincts. Fasting, poverty, celibacy, and self-denial were common practices because the spirit or soul, not the body, was important and needed refinement for salvation. **Scholasticism** was a product of medieval Catholic philosophers, most notably Thomas Aquinas. It attempted to reconcile Aristotelian realism with the teachings of the Catholic Church. Scholastics believed that truth was not only uncovered through the workings of the mind, but was also acquired with faith through the revelations of God. Bodily development through exercise and physical activity is important for the welfare of an individual, but it is secondary to one's spirituality.

Two philosophical approaches to education surfacing in the 1930s were **aritomism** and **essentialism.** The former is a combination of some of Aristotle's and Thomas Aquinas's principles, with the theological doctrine removed. While its goal is human happiness, it seeks absolute, unchanging truths that are universal for all people at all times. It is a philosophy of **dualism** in viewing the human body and mind as separate, with physical faculties subordinate to cognitive abilities. For the aritomist, physical education consists of a core of activities (though some local variation is allowed) and serves as a valuable antidote to demanding intellectual stimulation. Essentialism also subscribes to a basic core of knowledge, skills, and values inherent in physical performance activities that should be instilled in all learners. The essentialist favors a broad-based curriculum grounded in the liberal arts, stresses industriousness, and fosters self-discipline.

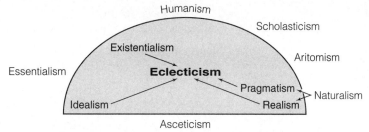

Figure 6.2 Traditional and contemporary philosophies.

ECLECTICISM

Very few humans are cut from the mold of any one particular philosophy. Most of us draw our ideas, thoughts, beliefs, and practices from two or more philosophies. More often than not, we draw upon a multitude of philosophies in eclectic fashion. Even though some consider **eclecticism** an unsystematic and incoherent approach toward philosophical conviction, it, nevertheless, helps learners resolve in their own minds some of the overriding confusion and conflict they find when attempting to untangle the threads of various philosophical traditions. As individuals grow intellectually and continue to study the discipline of philosophy, they may find eclecticism a useful stepping-stone toward acquiring a more unified approach in their personal philosophy.

WHAT IS A PERSONAL PHILOSOPHY?

Philosophy provides a basis for establishing a core of values and beliefs that guides an individual's conduct and approach to life. A **personal philosophy** is the sum of one's fundamental values, beliefs, attitudes, goals, objectives, criteria, and standards. It is a way of looking at life, the world, a career, or a profession. It is a credo that shapes actions. Molded by knowledge, ideas, experiences, social pressures, intuition, and reflection, one's personal philosophy will change just as one's position and status in life changes. If change is one of the constants in life, then one's personal philosophy is in a state of flux, often reflecting changes one undergoes in age, lifestyle, social status, and occupation.

One's occupation and profession have a great influence on one's personal philosophy. Because physical education subsumes physical activity, physical educators, by and large, lead an active lifestyle. Physical activity, thus, is an essential component of their personal philosophy, and it plays a vital role within their profession. In embracing physical activity, physical educators need to reconcile their own beliefs and practices with traditions and trends of their profession, thereby making it necessary for them to formulate a personal philosophy.

The Necessity of a Personal Philosophy

Personal philosophy guides behavior. This is critically important for physical educators who have the important responsibility of nurturing children and youth in physical activities from preschool through high school. Whether one's emphasis is wellness, fitness, movement fundamentals, sport skills, or leisure activities (and these will vary according to grade level), one's personal philosophy drives the way one presents information and the manner in which one broaches subject matter. Philosophy is important, not only in planning and teaching daily lessons, but also for curriculum development, teacher-pupil interaction, parent-teacher conferences, and departmental administration.

Constructing One's Own Personal Philosophy

With a basic understanding of traditional philosophies and the basic branches of philosophy, we are now in a position to undertake a preliminary identification and construction of our personal philosophy, our credo. A number of questions center on one's purpose in life and vocational preferences: Who am I? What do I want from life? What is my role? Why have I chosen a career in physical education and/or sport? What do I want from that career? Where do I want to go professionally? How will I get there?

To help students construct a personal philosophy that also relates to developing a philosophy of physical education, the following steps are offered:

First, examine the philosophies of various leaders and organizations within the profession for direction and guidance. For example, read the National Association for Sport and Physical Education's position statement about the components of quality physical education programs.

As a second step, analyze your own beliefs and experiences. In reflecting upon past experiences and their contribution to your personal philosophy as it relates to physical education and sport, consider the following:

- the attitude of parents toward physical education and sports
- parents' participation in physical activities
- grandparents' participation and values
- peer relationships
- cultural influences
- socioeconomic influences
- religious influences
- family leisure influences
- gender role models, especially regarding participation
- your family's health and lifestyles

Third, share your responses with others and listen to their responses. Compare your ideas with those of others. This is an opportunity to defend your ideas and determine the areas you need to reconsider or consider more carefully.

Physical educators need to contemplate the development of a philosophy in several different areas within physical education, especially as it relates to teaching and duties and responsibilities of teachers in the schools. Of high importance is the role of physical education as part of education in general. What physical activity and physical education offer students may give insight on the benefits of education in general. Teachers need to determine how they feel about students and the teacher's role in the lives of students. In addition to having a philosophy of their discipline, physical education teachers need a philosophy for evaluating pupils. In matters involving curriculum development, teachers need to consider their beliefs about how students learn and the relevance of attendance, dressing for class, and participation. They also need a plan for fostering collegiality among ethnically diverse groups. This list is by no means complete, but is offered to stimulate thoughts and ideas. Once a philosophy has taken shape, the teacher must reflect upon how it will affect his or her approach to education in general and physical education in particular. This philosophy will provide the framework necessary to guide the person's actions as an individual and in interactions with others.

ETHICAL ISSUES

As mentioned earlier in this chapter, the branch of philosophy called ethics is concerned with right and wrong, morality, and how individuals treat each other and themselves. Today, increasing pressure is placed upon educators and the schools to address all the issues and problems facing youth. This expanded role has included teaching students about drugs, alcohol, tobacco, HIV and AIDS, and moral and character development issues that were once thought to be the responsibility of parents. In teaching about moral issues, example is one of the best techniques. But in addressing moral issues, "right" and "wrong" are not always clearly delineated. Let's consider some situations.

Signing a Contract

Suppose a teacher signs a contract in early summer to begin teaching at a particular school in the fall. Later that same summer, a more appealing job at another school is advertised. Should the teacher pursue the other more desirable job and ask to be released from the contract already signed if a position is offered at another school?

When one signs a contract, one agrees to the terms and conditions laid out in the document. Breaking a contract is not only inconsiderate and unethical on the part of the violator, but it also reveals dishonesty. The violator places an undue hardship on the employer who entered into an agreement in good faith, but now has to search for an adequate replacement at the last minute. If a replacement with comparable credentials cannot be found, it may well deprive pupils of the quality education to which they are entitled. Moreover, breaking a contract could taint one as dishonest and untrustworthy, damaging one's reputation and reducing opportunities for career advancement later on. In this scenario, it's best to honor the contract and apply for other positions when it is appropriate to do so.

Calling in Sick

In addition to sick days, most school districts give teachers a certain number of personal leave days to handle emergencies or unexpected situations that may arise. Suppose a teacher who has already used up all of her personal leave days is tired and would rather do things other than go to school. She calls in sick and rationalizes the action by convincing herself that she works hard and is entitled to a day off. Is this behavior appropriate?

Certainly not! Sick days are provided for the specific purpose of allowing teachers time off to recover from acute illnesses—colds, fevers, flu, and the like. Sick days are also intended to help reduce the spread of respiratory infections by having healthy teachers in classrooms and other work areas. A teacher who abuses a school's sick-day policy is placing personal, selfish interests above the educational needs of the students. A substitute teacher will fill in, and many of them are quite capable, but continuity and valuable instruction time is lost, for no matter how qualified the substitute, time is squandered because the students and their routines are unfamiliar. In this case, the teacher needs to reevaluate her interest in teaching. Teachers must be passionate about teaching, and if they are passionate, they will use sick days only when they are really sick. They enthusiastically approach each day's experiences with their students. It takes dedication, motivation, and patience to be an effective teacher. Those who do not have these traits should consider another profession.

Use of School Copy Machine

A teacher uses the school copy machine to photocopy a personal letter for family members and friends. He does not pay for the copies, but instead justifies his action with the rationalization that his low teaching salary entitles him to such perquisites as personal photocopying. Why is his logic faulty and his behavior unscrupulous?

The teacher has been placed in a position of trust and has an obligation to honor that trust. Using a school copy machine for personal purposes, even for just one copy, is essentially stealing from the school and the taxpayers who financially support that school. The teacher should first determine if the school has a system of paying for personal copies made on the school copy machine. If there is no policy to reimburse the school for personal photocopying, he should find some other place to make personal copies rather than using the school copy machine.

Use of School Telephone

A teacher is frequently on the telephone during her planning period. Most of the calls are not related to school business. Some of the calls are long distance and are charged to the school telephone bill. What does this set of circumstances tell you about ethics and honesty?

Using the school telephone for personal long distance phone calls is very similar to using the school copy machine for making personal copies. The first part of the telephone/planning period scenario, however, is different. In this situation the teacher is using a planning period that has been provided to prepare for classes—developing lesson plans, constructing tests, grading papers, preparing materials for distribution, and completing other necessary tasks. The teacher is paid to be working during the planning periods. By neglecting to use planning period as designated, the teacher is stealing time from the school and—more importantly—shortchanging her pupils. Consequently, lessons might not be fully developed, feedback on papers and tests might be delayed, and handouts and other educational materials might not be prepared on time. To reemphasize, teachers must be dedicated and motivated. Misuse of the planning period shows how little concern this teacher has for her students.

"Throwing Out the Ball"

A physical education teacher begins a unit on basketball with an eighth-grade class. For the second lesson, he decides the morning news is more important than teaching basketball skills. Moreover, he believes everyone has played basketball and knows how to play the game anyway. When the class arrives, he divides the students into four teams and sets up two basketball games. He throws out a ball for each game and then retires into his office where he can read his newspaper and at the same time watch the two games through the observation window of his office. What does this circumstance tell you about this physical educator?

It is precisely this type of teacher who gives physical education a black eye. Physical education is more than just playing. Learning and developing sports skills, in this case, basketball, is one aspect of physical education. But even for an activity as popular as basketball, which many youngsters begin to play at an early age, formal instruction is needed, and that requires sound preparation and planning. Skills must be presented, drills must be set up, and practice opportunities must be provided. A teacher's throwing out the ball so that students can play a game does not automatically guarantee learning.

The physical educator who resorts to throwing out the ball is more than just plain lazy. He shirks his responsibility to educate his students. He robs them of much-needed learning experiences that emphasize skill development. He simply does not want to take the time to help his students learn. In terms of professional ethics, he is not carrying out his duties as a physical education teacher, and, morally, he is corrupting the system. This type of teacher, obviously, has no place in physical education.

Spending as Little Time as Possible at School

At a particular school, teachers are expected to arrive by 7:50 A.M. and stay until 3:30 P.M. One teacher there pulls into the parking lot each morning at 7:50 A.M. and leaves the gym office at 3:25 P.M., knowing it takes five minutes to walk to the parking lot and get into her car. What does this behavior tell you about the dedication and motivation of this teacher?

Even though this teacher is complying with school policy by spending the required hours each day on the school grounds, the teacher is sending a message to her students that shows she has little interest in education or in them. She is a typical clock watcher who can barely wait for quitting time to arrive. She tolerates the hours in order to receive a paycheck. Teaching is not a job in which employees punch a time clock. Pupils need teachers who care about them and who are willing to help them, no matter how much time it takes. A genuine teacher is dedicated, motivated, patient, and enthusiastic. The clock watcher has none of these traits and has no business in the teaching profession.

Other Issues

Many other ethical scenarios could be proposed—and do exist. These might include teaching a swimming class without a lifeguard present, timing students in the mile run on an exceptionally hot day, neglecting students with low fitness levels or poor skills, or just getting by in fulfilling responsibilities.

ETHICAL TRAITS AND CHARACTERISTICS

Reputable physical educators should model ethical and moral behavior. To acquire these traits, you must first identify what acceptable ethics (beliefs) and morals (behavior) are and then devise a strategy for adopting them. One strategy for inculcating good ethics and pursuing moral excellence includes recognizing and becoming aware of moral issues, respecting yourself, and loving your work.

Table 6.1 lists traits that promote good ethics and traits that promote bad ones. Prospective physical educators should evaluate their own ethical traits to determine in which category they fit best. Teachers who are most effective

Table 6.1 Contrasting Ethical Traits

TRAITS THAT PROMOTE GOOD ETHICS	TRAITS THAT PROMOTE BAD ETHICS
Self-control, rationality, an ability to gain some distance from an emotional event or issue	Recklessness, emotionalism, a tendency to act with emotion and self-interest
Honesty and integrity; an interest in achieving something of value	Drive and desire; an interest in succeeding by whatever means
A sense of fair play	A win-at-all-costs attitude
Patience, a willingness to wait for the right opportunity	Opportunism, a tendency to jump at the first attractive offer one receives
Constancy, singleness of purpose, the development of a life and career guided by clear values	Adaptability, vacillation, a tendency to adopt values that work or that are currently popular
Conscientiousness, thoroughness	Inefficiency, lack of productivity
Courage, a willingness to stand by one's values in the face of difficulty	Strategic shrewdness, an unwillingness to let extraneous values stand in the way of success
Altruism, a tendency to look out for the rights and interests of others	Survivalism, a tendency to take care of oneself and let others take care of their own problems

in reaching each pupil demonstrate traits that promote good ethics. For someone who does not demonstrate the traits that promote good ethics, a profession other than teaching is more appropriate.

CASE STUDIES INVOLVING ETHICS

Following are three case studies describing situations that have occurred in K–12 school settings. For each situation determine the issues involved and suggest a plan of action.

Confidentiality versus Legal Obligation

Brenda is an average student in the middle school. Miss Redding is her physical education teacher and basketball coach. Brenda feels comfortable talking with Miss Redding and often comes to her office just to chat. One day she wants to talk about something and the following conversation occurs.

Brenda says, "I need to talk to you about something but you have to promise not to tell anyone first."

"I promise."

"I was raped last night."

"Who did it?"

"I don't want to tell you. He will hurt me if I tell anyone."

"Have you called the police or seen a doctor?"

"No and I don't want to."

"Have you told your parents or anyone else?"

"No!"

"Brenda, you need to get some help, and we need to report this to the proper authorities."

"I don't want anyone else to know and you promised not to tell anyone." With that the bell rang and Brenda left for class.

What would you do?

Coaching Integrity

The Ballard eighth-grade girls' basketball team is playing its biggest rival, Vining. The game is close, and each team is playing well. A Ballard girl travels, and the ball is awarded to Vining on the side of the court. The game is played in a small gymnasium which does not have enough room for a player to throw the ball in bounds, so the court has a restraining line behind which a player must stand during the in-bounds play. The Vining player stands in the court but behind the restraining line to make the play, a maneuver that is clearly within the rules. The official nearest the play calls a violation on the Vining team and awards the ball to Ballard.

The Vining coach gets very upset and calls the official to the bench. The Ballard coach, who always carries a rules book, gets out the book and also approaches the bench. What should the Ballard coach do?

Access for All Students

A sixth-grade girl with cerebral palsy is confined to a wheelchair. Her upper-body strength is not very good. She is capable of moving herself around, but handling doors is impossible. Each day someone helps her get through the doors of the locker rooms so she can get ready for class;

then after class, someone opens the door so she can exit the locker room. One day, after a physical education class, she was in the locker room and ready to return to the classroom, but all the girls left without helping her leave the locker room. The teacher (a woman) did not check the locker room to make sure everyone was out. The child was in the locker room until the next class came in to get ready for physical education class, some ten minutes later. Discuss this situation.

On the Web

http://www.blackwellpublishers.co.uk/philos/
Philosophy Resources site contains a variety of links to general philosophy Internet sites. Includes a list of chat rooms and links to philosophy teaching tools.

http://www.ets.uidaho.edu/center_for_ethics
Home page for the University of Idaho Center for Ethics. Provides information about research being conducted and recommends books to read on sport ethics. Includes information on character education curriculum for K–12 programs.

http://www.utm.edu/research/iep/westtime.htm
Internet Encyclopedia of Philosophy; excellent source of information for Western philosophy from ancient times to the modern period.

http://www.friesian.com/#contents
Friesian School Web site; contains useful information on the history of philosophy.

http://www.cces.ca
Canadian Centre for Ethics in Sport provides information about programs such as the Spirit of Sport, Promoting Fair Play, and Achieving Drug-Free Sport.

http://www.iaps.net.
Web site of the International Association for the Philosophy of Sport. Contains information on books, conferences, and related resources.

Key Terms

aesthetics The branch of philosophy concerned with the appreciation of beauty, taste, and the quality of life (page 129).

aritomism A philosophical approach that seeks absolute, unchanging truths that are universal for all people at all times (page 134).

asceticism A belief and practice in which spiritual development is emphasized over bodily needs as a path to salvation (page 134).

axiology The branch of philosophy concerned with values (page 129).

dualism A belief in the separation of mind and body (page 134).

eclecticism In terms of personal philosophy, the acceptance of ideas, thoughts, beliefs, and practices from two or more philosophical approaches (page 135).

epistemology The branch of philosophy that deals with the acquisition of knowledge (page 128).

essentialism A belief in a basic core of knowledge, skills, and values that should be instilled in all learners (page 134).

ethics A dimension of axiology that deals with moral judgments, questions of how individuals treat each other and themselves (page 129).

existentialism A modern philosophy based on the absurdity of life and knowing the inner self. It predicates freedom of choice and the need to accept responsibility for one's own life in order to become the best one can become (page 132).

humanism A philosophy that emphasizes the value of the human being and the power of human intelligence as well as appreciation and respect for the human body (page 133).

idealism The traditional philosophy in which only ideas are real, and the world of the material is not real (page 130).

logic The branch of philosophy that involves the use of thought processes and reasoning power to reach correct conclusions (page 129).

metaphysics The branch of philosophy that is concerned with the nature of reality—questions about mind and body, the existence of God, and the nature of being, among others (page 128).

naturalism The oldest philosophy, which holds that all truth and reality are found in the laws of nature and material things; it denies the supernatural (page 134).

personal philosophy The sum of one's fundamental values, beliefs, attitudes, goals, objectives, criteria, and standards; one's personal philosophy shapes one's actions (page 135).

philosophy An academic discipline; also any one of various established or traditional ways of looking at the world (such as idealism or existentialism) that have been defined and identified by those who practice the discipline, whether in the academy or not (page 128).

pragmatism A modern philosophy which holds that experience is the only source of truth and that what experience teaches is valuable only if it has practical applications and helps people achieve their goals (page 132).

realism The traditional philosophy, opposed to idealism, which holds that things do exist independently of the human mind (page 130).

Scholasticism Christian philosophy of the Middle Ages that stressed analysis of the Bible and other religious writings; faith was built on the revealed word of God and the wisdom of Christian thinkers (page 134).

Multiple Choice Questions

1. Philosophy is
   a. a review of a person's past experiences
   b. a series of questions for the gaining of factual knowledge
   c. a set of values and beliefs that guides individual conduct
   d. a study of how the body performs under stress
   e. sum of beliefs, values, and attitudes

2. The traditional philosophy in which the material world is not real is
   a. naturalism
   b. idealism
   c. pragmatism
   d. existentialism
   e. realism

3. A modern philosophy that holds that experience is the only source of truth is known as
   a. naturalism
   b. idealism
   c. pragmatism
   d. existentialism
   e. realism

4. The branch of philosophy that is concerned with the nature of reality is
   a. metaphysics
   b. ethics
   c. aesthetics
   d. axiology
   e. epistemology

5. The study of the acquisition of knowledge is called
   a. metaphysics
   b. ethics
   c. aesthetics
   d. axiology
   e. epistemology

6. The philosophical approach that deals with moral judgments and how individuals treat each other and themselves is known as
   a. metaphysics

b. ethics
c. aesthetics
d. axiology
e. epistemology

7. The sum of one's fundamental values, beliefs, attitudes, goals, objectives, criteria, and standards is

a. epistemology
b. philosophy
c. personal philosophy
d. aritomism
e. essentialism

8. Which of the following does *not* need to be considered when analyzing your own feelings and experiences in preparation for writing your personal philosophy of physical education and sport?

a. grandparents' participation in sport
b. world politics
c. religious influences
d. cultural influences
e. peer relationships

9. In constructing their own personal philosophy, students should

a. examine the philosophies of leaders in the profession
b. analyze their own beliefs and experiences
c. compare their own ideas with those of others
d. a and b of the above
e. a, b, and c of the above

10. The philosophical dimension that is concerned with beauty, taste, and quality of life is

a. metaphysics
b. axiology
c. aesthetics
d. ethics
e. epistemology

Critical Thinking Questions

1. Mr. Rodriquez and Ms. Jones are two physical education teachers assigned to teach a large volleyball class together. As they discuss their plans for the volleyball unit, Mr. Rodriquez indicates that he wants to give the students a skills test the first day of class to measure their ability and then assign them to groups according to their abilities. Ms. Jones disagrees. On the first day she prefers to go over the rules and get the students involved in playing the game because she believes doing so will enhance their self-development. On the

basis of each teacher's approach to beginning this volleyball class, discuss the philosophical leanings of each one and give your reasons for classifying each teacher the way you did.

2. Jennifer is a student in Mr. Chen's physical education class, which has been learning badminton over the past month. One day after a participating in several rigorous drills, Jennifer approached Mr. Chen and complained about all the hard work he had put them through during the class. In response, Mr. Chen stated that experience is the best teacher and that the varied experiences of the drills and practices would give her a greater opportunity for mastering badminton. From a philosophical standpoint, how would you classify Mr. Chen and why?

3. Mr. Smiley, one of the physical education teachers at Central High School, also serves as the basketball coach. On the morning after a one-point loss to Central's fiercest rival, East End, Billy, a student in Mr. Smiley's first period class, asked the coach why he notified the official of a scorekeeper's error that would have kept his best player in the game after he committed his fifth personal, or disqualifying, foul. Mr. Smiley said he was from the old school where honesty and sportsmanship meant something. From your knowledge of traditional philosophies, how would you classify Mr. Smiley's behavior, and explain whether it would have been morally wrong for Mr. Smiley to allow his best player to continue playing with five personal fouls.

4. Cara and Leung, undergraduate physical education majors in Dr. Lopez's History and Philosophy of Sport and Physical Education class, are confused by Dr. Lopez's remarks in today's class. She was emphatic about the shortcomings of eclecticism when she stated that students often take the easy way out by classifying themselves as eclectics because they believe they have traces of each traditional and modern philosophy embedded in their own philosophical leanings. Cara, a volleyball player, thought she was an eclectic leaning toward pragmatism, while Leung, although she believes in the self-realization of existentialism, contends that existentialism is only one facet of her philosophical belief system. What advice can you give to Cara and Leung regarding their philosophical orientations? Analyze Dr. Lopez's assessment of eclecticism.

5. Jerry, a physical education teacher at Conklin Elementary School, is enthusiastic about teaching physical education and his choice of activities shows it. He offers units in adventure education that emphasize cooperation, trust building, and confidence development. Whenever possible, Jerry tries to measure achievement and improvement in these areas. Jerry's principal maintains that Jerry is an idealist, but Jerry insists that he is a realist. Who is correct and why?

Notes and References

Harrison, J. M., Blakemore, C. L., and Buck, M. M. *Instructional Strategies for Secondary School Physical Education,* 5th ed. Dubuque, Iowa: McGraw-Hill, 2001.

Howard, B. K., and Howard, M. R. "What a Difference a Choice Makes!" Strategies, 10, no. 3 (1997): 16–20.

Kretchmar, R. S. *Practical Philosophy of Sport.* Champaign, Ill: Human Kinetics, 1994.

Lottes, C. R. "Action Plan for Fitness," *Strategies,* 10, no. 3 (1997): 27–32.

Solomon, G. B. "Fair Play in the Gymnasium: Improving Social Skills among Elementary School Students," *The Journal of Physical Education, Recreation and Dance,* 68, no. 5 (1997): 22–25.

Spencer, A. F. "Ethics in Physical and Sport Education," *The Journal of Physical Education, Recreation and Dance,* 67, no. 7 (1996): 37–39.

Strean, W. B. "Ideology Critique: Improving Instruction by Thinking about Your Thinking," *The Journal of Physical Education, Recreation and Dance,* 68, no. 4 (1997): 53–56.

7

PHYSICAL EDUCATION AS AN ACADEMIC DISCIPLINE

Chapter Objectives

After reading this chapter, the student will be able to

- Define what is meant by an academic discipline

- Define and describe the core content knowledge area of physical education

- Identify and describe the subject matter of the core content knowledge areas of physical education

- Describe the role and function of pedagogy courses in the preparation of physical education teachers

- Identify and define at least three allied areas of specialization that have emerged from physical education

Physical education is predicated upon physical activity and human movement. Consequently, the body of knowledge that forms this **academic discipline** is broad-based, drawing heavily from anatomy, physiology, physics, biochemistry, nutrition, psychology, and sociology. In the twenty-first century, the concept of "wellness" tends to subsume physical education and limit it to a single physical fitness spoke on the wellness wheel that includes optimal emotional, intellectual, social, and spiritual fitness. But wellness—that is, total well-being—need not necessarily subsume physical education; instead, wellness can be and often is recognized as a legitimate outcome of physical education.

Because the human body is so instrumental in the processes of physical activity and human movement, a knowledge and understanding of human anatomy and physiology is essential to the teacher of physical education. For teaching, analyzing, and evaluating fitness, the physical educator must have a clear understanding and working knowledge of the skeletal, muscular, cardiovascular, respiratory, circulatory, nervous, and endocrine systems. A physical education teacher must be able to explain how the human body responds to exercise and must be able to use principles of exercise physiology in applied settings. A teacher of physical education must have sufficient knowledge of nutrition and biochemistry to understand the influence of caloric intake and energy expenditure on the human body. In teaching movement fundamentals and sport skills, the physical educator must understand movement patterns—an understanding that is normally gained through knowledge of developmental psychology, motor behavior, and biomechanics.

In sum, then, a physical educator must have a thorough understanding and working knowledge of human movement, human physiology, body mechanics, and motor behavior. In addition, the teacher must have sufficient preparation in **pedagogy** to transmit content knowledge effectively to students. The instructor must also have preparation in adapted (or special) physical education in order to reach physically and mentally challenged students. Finally, the physical educator needs at least minimal exposure to the allied specialization areas of athletic training, sports management, exercise gerontology, and health promotion. All of these areas contribute to the broad perspective of knowledge that constitutes physical education. This chapter has a threefold purpose. First, it will examine the **core content knowledge** of a course of study in physical education, which consists of classes in or related to the sciences, social sciences, and humanities. Next it will survey pedagogical knowledge covered by classes in methods of teaching. Lastly, it will introduce the allied areas of specialization related to physical education.

CORE CONTENT KNOWLEDGE

Anatomy and Physiology

Physical education is based on knowledge of anatomy and physiology—knowledge of the human body. In particular, physical education teachers need to know how muscles function and what actions they perform. They need to know about the heart and the circulation of blood; about the lungs, respiration, and the exchange of oxygen and carbon dioxide; about the nervous system and sensory and motor impulses; about the endocrine system and the role of hormones during exercise and rest. Knowledge of these and other bodily systems and their functions give physical educators a clearer understanding of human movement, exercise, and skill acquisition for physical performance.

Physiology of Exercise

The study of physiology of exercise leads to understanding how the body responds to exercise. This knowledge area provides substantive information for developing and maintaining effective but safe levels of physical fitness and for increasing our knowledge about the benefits of exercise. It deals with virtually every system of the human body in determining how it responds to the stress of exercise.

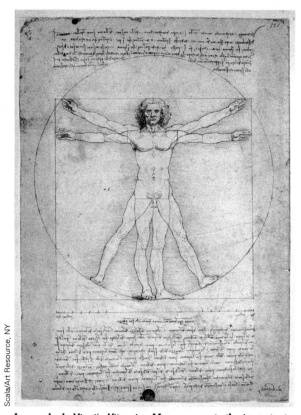

Scala/Art Resource, NY

Leonardo da Vinci's *Vitruvian Man* represents the important relationship between anatomy/physiology and physical education.

Exercise physiology includes the study of cardiovascular endurance or aerobic (with oxygen) activity in which the body can exercise for a long period of time at less than a maximum effort (for example, a five-kilometer run); anaerobic (without oxygen) activity in which maximum or near maximum efforts can be sustained for a short period of time (100-meter dash); muscular strength, the maximum amount an individual can lift; muscular endurance, the ability to sustain a less-than-maximum effort for a long period of time; and flexibility, the ability of the body to bend and stretch.

Physiological information is also useful for diet and weight control, understanding the safe temperatures and

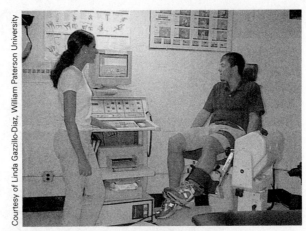

Future physical educators get hands-on laboratory experience in physiology of exercise and biomechanics.

environmental conditions for exercise, overcoming certain physical disabilities, and coping with chronic diseases, such as diabetes and coronary artery disease.

Biomechanics

The discipline of **biomechanics** uses principles of physics to analyze motion, force, leverage, friction, momentum, velocity, and other physical variables involving human movement. Biomechanics exposes the prospective physical educator to motion analyses of such fundamental movements as walking, running, throwing, striking, and kicking that are necessary for the performance of physical skills. It helps teachers analyze the movement or skill themselves by breaking it down into meaningful parts. Instructors can then present the parts of a skill to their students in a progressive sequence, encouraging them to master one part at a time. When all parts are mastered, the student will have a good grasp of performing the entire skill successfully. In addition to its usefulness for teachers in helping beginners to master basic physical skills, biomechanical principles enable physical educators to provide advice to advanced learners who want to raise their skill level and to physically disabled learners who need assistance in performing rudimentary motor movements.

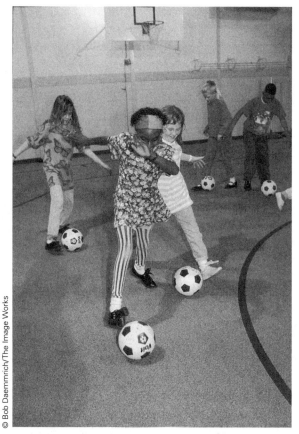

© Bob Daemmrich/The Image Works

Elementary school pupils engaged in learning basic locomotor activities.

Motor Behavior

Motor learning, motor development, and motor control, three components of **motor behavior,** provide the prospective physical educator with the neuromuscular basis for comprehending movement patterns and teaching physical skills. **Motor learning** is the most useful for teachers because it deals with changes in the performance of physical skills. Physical educators can apply principles of practice, feedback, hand-eye coordination, reaction time, and agility to teaching fundamental movements and physical skills to pupils at different skill levels. The area of **motor development** is an outgrowth of developmental psychology in that it looks at skill acquisition and performance at various developmental stages of the individual—initially in infancy and early childhood but now through all stages of the human life span. Although knowledge from this area is most useful to physical educators who teach at preschools and elementary schools, in recent decades it has been valuable for exercise leaders who work with older adults. **Motor control,** the newest member of this triad, focuses on the mental processes behind motor and physical skill acquisition and performance. This discipline offers physical educators valuable assistance in teaching, developing, and evaluating motor and physical skill acquisition by helping them understand neuromuscular responses to cognitive function.

Sport and Exercise Psychology

The discipline of **sport psychology** has expanded to include **exercise psychology** because physical educators have recognized the need to study psychology as it relates to exercise and exercise adherence as well as to sport. Sport psychology is the study of psychological and behavioral issues as they relate to sport. This content area includes personality types and determinants, concentration, self-concept, motivation, self-efficacy, aggression, anxiety, and competition. While some of the information, particularly that involving motivation, self-concept, and anxiety, is useful to physical education teachers, a great deal of it is even more valuable to coaches of athletic teams in applied settings at all levels.

In recent years, however, emphasis in sport psychology has shifted to exercise adherence in an attempt to reach a broad audience to inform them about the importance of undertaking and maintaining an exercise program for a lifetime. With exercise adherence, motivation is the key to keeping people involved, and this has great implications for physical educators. As the incidence of childhood obesity continues to rise and the constant attraction or addiction to video games reinforces a sedentary lifestyle, physical educators need to motivate young people to undertake and maintain an active lifestyle. Principles of motivation, self-concept, and self-efficacy covered in sport psychology are especially useful. For adherence to be lasting, motivation must be intrinsic, and teachers schooled in psychological techniques might use the notions of self-concept and self-efficacy (performing a given task successfully) to inculcate and reinforce intrinsic motivation.

Sport Sociology

The discipline of **sport sociology** studies the structure and patterns of social organizations and the dynamics of groups participating in sports. On a general level, it can deal with the effects of sport on a particular culture or the development of sport within a culture, while in a more restricted setting, it might involve spectator violence, crowd behavior, ethnic or gender discrimination, or social benefits of regular physical activity. Sport also is connected to religion, politics, education, the economy, mass media, and opportunities for girls and women in sport as participants, coaches, and administrators.

The value of sport sociology for physical educators lies in group dynamics and equality issues for minorities and women. Concern about gender equality has been fueled by Title IX of the Educational Amendments Act of 1972. Title IX stipulated that all programs receiving federal funding must comply with its provisions, which called for equal representation and equal spending for both genders. As a result, physical education teachers must insure that boys and girls receive equal opportunities when participating in physical education classes.

Sport History

As a core content area, **sport history** enables teachers of physical education to discover their profession's heritage and how and why physical education has developed into what it is today. It gives them knowledge about and insight into the leaders and pioneers of their profession, some of whom may serve as role models for them. It also provides them with background information about the sporting activities they often teach. Knowledge of history is useful in pointing out the mistakes of the past and helping ensure that educators today do not repeat those mistakes.

Sport Philosophy

Sport philosophy, among other things, brings values and ethics to teachers to help govern their behavior and their interaction with pupils, administrators, and parents. It is also valuable for athletic coaches who use its principles for developing a behavior code among their athletes and for adopting team rules and regulations. On the personal level, it helps physical educators formulate their own philosophy about movement, exercise, and skill acquisition and how they might go about teaching those topics.

PEDAGOGICAL KNOWLEDGE

Pedagogy

Foremost, physical educators are teachers. Although their emphasis is physical activity and human movement, physical educators impart knowledge that helps their students to grow emotionally, socially, and intellectually as well as physically. The core content knowledge area that prepares physical educators to disseminate information and nurture the learner is pedagogy, the study of teaching, which involves the curriculum and instructional methods. In recent years, a new term, **sport pedagogy,** has been introduced into the American education lexicon. International in scope, sport pedagogy not only includes physical education methodologies and curriculum development in the school setting, but also encompasses teaching sports skills and coaching athletic teams in communities, clubs, and other organizations outside of schools. Because a substantial number of physical education teachers coach athletic teams, coaches will find much of the instructional methodology of physical education applicable in athletic environments.

In recent years with increased interest in pedagogical research, the content area of sport pedagogy has expanded to include curricular and instructional issues and multiple teaching strategies. Research in sport pedagogy began in earnest in the 1970s. Prior to that time, very little research

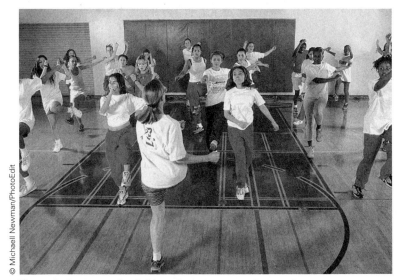

Physical educators, schooled in pedagogy, practice their craft in a high school physical education class.

had been conducted on curriculum and instruction issues as they relate to general sport pedagogy. Now, over thirty years later, much more is known about effective teaching and an effective teaching environment. Research in this area, for example, investigates and assesses effective teaching strategies, the interactions of students and teachers, and instructional materials. Early on, research focused on current teaching practices and the effects of various modifications of those practices. Now research examines the context in which the teaching occurs—for example, developing effective physical education lessons for large classes in an urban environment with limited space. The last thirty years have also seen the development of curriculum models dealing with fitness, sport education, and adventure education, and such teaching styles as command (teacher-directed learning), reciprocal (student partnership learning), and guided discovery (teacher-assisted learning).

Adapted Physical Education

The content area of **adapted physical education** has been a part of the physical education curriculum since mid-century, but in recent decades the trend of mainstreaming students with disabilities (physical and mental) into regular physical education classes has made the basic adapted physical education course an essential component of every physical educator's undergraduate preparation. Then, in the 1970s, in the spirit of diversification, a number of undergraduate and graduate programs made it possible for students to complement their physical education certification with a concentration in adapted physical education. In this specialty, future physical educators learn to work with and help pupils who are confronted with physical and mental challenges, orthopedic conditions, perceptual impairment, and/or emotional instability.

ALLIED AREAS OF SPECIALIZATION

During the 1970s when a dearth of teaching positions in physical education kept young, energetic, and highly qualified physical educators in the unemployment line, physical education programs began to diversify, leading to the creation of several **allied areas of specialization,** or subdisciplines. One of the first allied specializations to emerge was athletic training, followed by sports management, exercise science, exercise gerontology, and health promotion, but in recent years athletic training, sports management, and exercise science have begun to establish separate baccalaureate programs with their own pool of degree candidates.

Athletic Training

The subdiscipline of **athletic training** deals with the prevention and rehabilitation of athletic injuries. Trainers can ill afford to err in assessing athletic injuries, so their preparation requires a thorough immersion in anatomy and physiology; this includes gross (cadaver) anatomy at some institutions, plus a cadre of courses in modalities, assessment, therapeutic exercise, clinical internships, and fieldwork. More often than not, athletic trainers in public schools need to be certified teachers, and the preferred certification of most trainers is physical education. Physical educators, too, can benefit from an introductory course in athletic training that normally covers prevention and care of most injuries common to physical education classes.

Sports Management

In the 1970s, **sports management** emerged to fill the void created by the scarcity of teaching positions. In this allied specialization, one follows a business-oriented curriculum to prepare for an administrative post at either the professional, semiprofessional, or collegiate level of sports. Although a course in management principles can be useful for physical educators who also coach athletic teams, it provides even greater benefits later on to the teacher who serves as department head or a coach who becomes an athletic director.

Exercise Science

Along with athletic training and sports management, exercise science emerged during the 1970s as physical education departments scrambled to find viable career options for students who abruptly discovered that the door to teaching and coaching had virtually closed. With a background in exercise physiology, students with a few advanced courses in physiology of exercise, exercise stress testing, and cardiac rehabilitation found employment in health spas, community centers, and private agencies (YMCAs AND YWCAs), hospitals, or corporate settings. Exercise science concentrations enabled students to explore and enter career paths they never thought were possible.

Exercise Gerontology

Through **exercise gerontology,** physical education attempts to reach people throughout their entire life span by combining principles of exercise with tenets and theories of aging. Like the other allied specializations, exercise gerontology was also a product of the 1970s and offered prospective physical education teachers another career option.

Health Promotion

The goal of **health promotion** is optimal health for people of all ages—sound physical, emotional, social, spiritual, and intellectual health, or what is termed wellness. Health promoters, whether physical educators or health educators, attempt to facilitate changes in lifestyle toward optimal health by enhancing awareness and changing behavior, as well as creating environments that support good health practices. Included within the physical area are fitness, nutrition, medical self-care, and substance-abuse control. The emotional dimension deals with stress management and coping with emotional crises. The social area involves communication with all peoples from every walk of life. Intellectual health stresses educational achievement and career development, while the spiritual is concerned with love, hope, and humanitarianism.

On the Web

http://www.acsm.org
The official home page of the American College of Sports Medicine. The site includes information about the organization, membership, conferences, grants, and other resources. It also contains information about certification examinations for exercise specialists and program directors.

www.EducationIndex.com/physed/
Contains list of Web sites with information and resources for physical education.

http://www.pecentral.com
An excellent Web site sponsored by Flaghouse Corporation, a manufacturer of physical education equipment. The site provides information on creative lessons, assessment, professional activities, current research, and instructional resources.

http://www.psyc.unt.edu/apadiv47
This site provides information about the profession of sport psychology, current trends, and significant issues. It also lists ways in which students can get involved.

http://www.aaasponline.org
Official home page of the Association for the Advancement of Applied Sport Psychology; it provides information about sport psychology, including conferences and resources as well as additional links.

http://www.nata.org
Official Web site of the National Athletic Trainers' Association. Includes information about membership, curriculum programs, certification examination, conferences, resources, and other links.

http://www.unb.ca/web/sportmanagement/nassm.htm
Official Web site of the North American Society for Sport Management.
Contains information on conferences, university programs, resources in
sport management, and links to other relevant sites.

http://www.healthpromotionjournal.com/publications/journal.htm
Site of American Journal of Health Promotion. Contains information on
trends and developments in health promotion.

http://www.ches.ua.edu/online/health/wang/
Contains articles from American Journal of Health Studies that can be
downloaded.

Key Terms

academic discipline The body of knowledge that constitutes a subject
area; physical education, social studies, or mathematics, for example
(page 152).

adapted physical education Strives to provide equal opportunities for
everyone—including those with disabilities—to participate in physical
activity and sport (page 160).

allied areas of specialization Initially, career options for physical education students who witnessed a great decline in teaching positions during
the 1970s. Now these specializations, such as athletic training and sports
management, have become degree programs that attract their own pool
of students (page 161).

athletic training Deals with the prevention, treatment, and rehabilitation of injuries that result from physical activity and athletic
competition (page 161).

biomechanics The study and analysis of the mechanics of human movement, with efficient movement as a goal (page 155).

core content knowledge A set of crucial (or core) courses that represent
the body of knowledge of a given discipline. In physical education, core
content courses are anatomy and physiology, physiology of exercise, biomechanics, motor behavior, psychology and sociology of sport, history
and philosophy of the discipline and profession (page 153).

exercise gerontology The combination of exercise physiology principles
with theories of aging in order to help older adults maintain their independence and a decent quality of life (page 162).

exercise physiology The study of the human body's response to exercise and physical activity (page 154).

exercise psychology The study of psychology as it relates to exercise
and motivation to continue to exercise on a regular basis (page 157).

health promotion An allied area of specialization whose focus is to help people attain optimal health, or wellness, through behavioral changes (page 162).

motor behavior Broad-based term that denotes the neuromuscular basis for movement patterns in performing physical skills; it includes motor control, motor development, and motor learning (page 156).

motor control The mental processes involved in the performance of motor and physical performance skills (page 157).

motor development The growth and development of the body in relationship to the acquisition of movement skills (page 156).

motor learning Motor-skill acquisition and changes in performance of physical skills (page 156).

pedagogy The study of teaching that involves the curriculum and instructional methods (page 152).

sport history The study and use of history to discover the heritage of physical education, background information of sporting activities, and the role and impact to physical activity at various points in time (page 158).

sport pedagogy A term with international meaning in that physical education methodologies and curriculum development are applied beyond the school setting to organizations, athletic teams, and sports clubs in the community (page 159).

sport psychology The study of psychological and behavioral issues as they relate to sport (page 157).

sport sociology The study of the structure and patterns of social organizations and the dynamics of groups participating in sport (page 158).

sports management An allied specialization program that involves the business aspects of sport, especially such areas as promotion, marketing, public relations, and finance. Graduates of sports management programs work as administrators and assistant administrators for professional sports teams and leagues as well as colleges and universities (page 162).

Multiple Choice Questions

1. Core content knowledge of physical education includes all of the following *except*
   a. anatomy and physiology
   b. physiology of exercise
   c. biomechanics
   d. mass communication
   e. motor behavior

2. The study of how the human body responds to exercise is

   a. elementary statistics
   b. sport sociology
   c. sport history
   d. biomechanics
   e. physiology of exercise

3. The study of motor-skill acquisition and changes in the performance of physical skills is

   a. motor control
   b. motor development
   c. motor learning
   d. sport pedagogy
   e. athletic training

4. The discipline that studies the prevention, treatment, and rehabilitation of injuries that may have occurred during physical activity is

   a. adapted physical education
   b. athletic training
   c. biomechanics
   d. exercise physiology
   e. motor learning

5. The discipline that studies the structure and patterns of social organizations and group dynamics is

   a. sport management
   b. sport pedagogy
   c. sport psychology
   d. sport sociology
   e. sport history

6. Bringing physical education methodologies to community sports programs is known as

   a. motor development
   b. motor learning
   c. motor control
   d. sport psychology
   e. sport pedagogy

7. The study of psychological and behavioral issues as they relate to sport is

   a. sport psychology
   b. sport sociology
   c. sport history
   d. sport philosophy
   e. sports management

8. Efficient human movement is the goal of

   a. sports management
   b. biomechanics
   c. sport sociology
   d. athletic training
   e. sport psychology

9. The goal of health promotion is

   a. unlimited health
   b. optimal health
   c. social health
   d. convenient health
   e. charitable health

10. The combination of exercise principles and theories of aging has opened up an area of service called

    a. exercise pediatrics
    b. exercise gerontology
    c. athletic training
    d. sports management
    e. aerobic dance

Critical Thinking Questions

1. Why is anatomy and physiology so important to the preparation of physical education majors that it is considered a core content knowledge course even though at most universities it is taught by faculty outside of the physical education department?

2. Exercise physiology, biomechanics, and motor behavior build upon the foundation laid in anatomy and physiology to form the scientific basis of physical education's knowledge core. What is the rationale for including sport psychology, sport sociology, sport history, and sport philosophy in the core content knowledge area?

3. Pedagogy, in its broadest sense, is the study of teaching, and the methodologies and curriculum development covered in these courses are instrumental for preparing prospective physical education teachers to become effective teachers. If pedagogy is so important in the preparation of physical education teachers, why is it separated from the other core content knowledge courses? Argue convincingly either for its inclusion in the core content knowledge area or for its permanent status outside of the core.

4. Athletic training and sports management have evolved from allied areas of specialization into separate and autonomous academic disciplines at most colleges and universities. Why is it important for

prospective physical education teachers to have exposure to both of these relatively new disciplines through their basic courses.

5. Traditional teacher preparation programs in physical education prepare students to work with students, K–12. The advent of concentrations in exercise physiology and exercise gerontology provide students with the knowledge and tools to work with adults in all age groups. Should physical education majors be required to take additional courses so they are qualified to work with all ages of the adult population, or is that best left to the exercise physiology specialist who has no background in pedagogy? Be sure to justify your answer.

References

American Journal of Health Promotion Web site. 2001. www.healthpromotionjournal.com.

Anshel, M. H. *Sport Psychology: From Theory to Practice,* 2d ed. Scottsdale, Ariz.: Gorsuch Scarisbrick, 1994.

Cox, R. H. *Sport Psychology: Concepts and Applications,* 4th ed. Dubuque, Iowa: Brown & Benchmark, 1998.

Eitzen, D. S. *Sport in Contemporary Society: An Anthology,* 4th ed. New York: St. Martin's, 1993.

Eitzen, D. S., and Sage, G. H. *Sociology of American Sport,* 7th ed. Dubuque, Iowa: Wm. C. Brown, 2003.

Harrison, J. M., Blakemore, C. L., and Buck, M. M. *Instructional Strategies for Secondary School Physical Education,* 5th ed. Dubuque, Iowa: McGraw-Hill, 2001.

Mosston, M., and Ashworth, S. *Teaching Physical Education,* 4th ed. New York: Macmillan, 1994.

Siedentop, D. *Introduction to Physical Education, Fitness, and Sport.* 5th ed. New York: McGraw-Hill, 2003.

Wuest, D. A., and Bucher, C. A. *Foundations of Physical Education and Sport,* 14th ed. Dubuque, Iowa: WCB McGraw-Hill, 2003.

8

PHYSICAL EDUCATION AS A PROFESSION

Chapter Objectives

After reading this chapter, the student will be able to

- Define the term *profession*
- Discuss the role of physical education in education
- Describe the roles and responsibilities of physical education teachers
- Explain the relationship of teaching physical education and professional organizations
- Identify at least three rewards and three challenges of teaching physical education
- Describe the responsibilities and challenges of coaching
- Describe career options in fitness, sport, and recreation
- Discuss factors that may influence one's choice of career

Physical education plays a significant role in the process of developing the whole child—that is, the mind and the body. Through the enhancement of the pupil's physical attributes, physical educators contribute to the learner's intellectual, emotional, and social growth and maturation. Physical education's multifaceted contributions stem from its foundation in the sciences, social sciences, and humanities (see Chapters 6 and 7). This diversity enables physical educators to function effectively within and outside of the educational arena. This chapter explores avenues of professional growth for someone with preparation in physical education.

THE TEACHING PROFESSION

A **profession** is an occupation that involves specific training and requires a demonstrated level of expertise and competence. The legal and medical professions, for instance, require years of highly specified training followed by a licensing procedure that verifies competence in these professions. In order to practice law, attorneys must first demonstrate their knowledge and competency on a bar exam; in order to practice medicine, physicians must meet internship and residency requirements before obtaining a medical license from the board of medical examiners in the state where they wish to practice.

Just as law and medicine have a set of standards required for entry into those fields, so, too does the profession of teaching. To enter the teaching profession, an individual must have a bachelor's degree (with a major in education or in the subject area to be taught), plus **certification,** or a license from the state in which one wishes to teach. Certification requirements are determined by each state and may vary widely from state to state. Some states will grant certification to an individual with a bachelor's degree in an education field from an accredited institution. Others require an examination plus the baccalaureate degree for a teaching license. Most states require a passing score on the PRAXIS, formerly the National Teacher's Examination, while some states construct their own examination.

In recent years, many colleges and universities have begun to require a five-year or master's degree program as a criterion for recommending an individual for admission to the teaching profession. Some states are also moving toward a model in which an individual is required to teach for two years under direct supervision of a mentor (an experienced teacher) prior to receiving certification.

PHYSICAL EDUCATION AS A TEACHING PROFESSION

Traditionally, careers in physical education and sport have focused on teaching and coaching in schools, colleges, or universities. Physical education teachers are hired to provide a service to their students by helping them improve their physical performance skills, fitness level, knowledge of sports and games, concepts about fitness and exercise, and understanding of themselves and others. Teachers in this profession use physical education's natural laboratory to foster cooperation and teamwork among their students.

Physical education teachers earn an undergraduate degree and, in some instances, a graduate degree in physical education. They must also meet other licensing requirements prior to receiving a teaching license. On the national level, the National Association for Sport and Physical Education (NASPE) has developed standards for beginning teachers that numerous states have adopted to guide them in their development of standards for judging the qualifications of beginning teachers.

A high percentage of physical educators also become coaches of athletic teams, giving them a dual role to perform in teaching and coaching. Teacher/coaches are held to a higher standard because of the influence they have on the lives of their students and athletes. One teacher who taught both physical education and health and also coached discovered that some students were with her for as many as five hours a day. That was more time than some parents spent with their children. Teaching often bears heavy responsibilities.

Physical educators are expected to exemplify high standards of physical fitness and to be strong models of sound

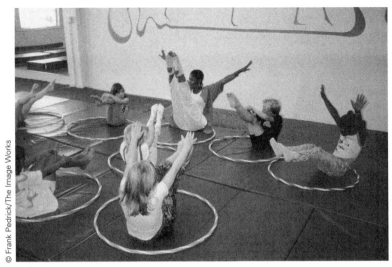

Health-conscious and robust physical educators will continue to move physical education forward.

general health practices. Physical educators who do not practice what they teach are not as effective as they would be if they demonstrated exemplary behavior. A physical educator who smokes, for example, is not as good a model of sound health practices for the profession or for students as is a teacher who does not smoke. Another reason to be physically fit is that a physical education instructor has to be physically active several hours of the day, teaching and demonstrating activities and exercises. Like all teachers, those who teach physical education must expend considerable physical energy, in addition to comparable amounts of emotional and mental energy, every day. Students who have physical education during the last period of the day deserve the same enthusiasm and energy from their physical education teachers as the students who take the class during the first period in the morning. Maintaining a degree of freshness requires a high degree of physical fitness on the part of the physical education teacher.

Consider also that the physical educator is most likely to be the resident fitness expert among the teachers, administrators, and staff in a school. As such, a physical education teacher has an opportunity to contribute to the well-being and fitness of colleagues as well as students. A staff that is physically fit will interact with students and teach more vibrantly and energetically—perhaps with more intellectual vigor and enthusiasm—than will a staff that is tired, ill, and under stress. So, as a professional, a physical education teacher can contribute to the health and well-being of fellow professionals by offering advice and perhaps even arranging teacher/staff wellness programs that would contribute to the overall performance of the school community.

THE IMPORTANCE OF PROFESSIONAL PHYSICAL EDUCATION

Professionals in physical education make major contributions to personal and community health and total well-being. Physical educators teach individuals about the importance of physical fitness and how to improve and maintain appropriate fitness levels. They also teach conditioning and sports skills that will enable people to participate in enjoyable physical activities throughout a lifetime. Beyond that, practicing what is taught about fitness and **wellness** in physical education classes may decrease an individual's risk of having a heart attack, stroke, or other life-threatening conditions. Furthermore, in health classes, physical educators focus on issues such as human sexuality, AIDS, tobacco and alcohol use, and the effects of other illegal drugs. An understanding of these topics could prevent unfortunate health consequences.

Physical education teachers find themselves in a unique position to gain valuable and helpful information about students. For instance, the physical education teacher observes students engaged in physical activities that often have major social and behavioral components. This perspective provides opportunities to supply information about students' social skills and interactions with other students. Many of these social and personal dynamics and characteristics may not be observable in other classroom settings. This knowledge can be beneficial in the overall efforts of the school to help each student, especially those who may have learning disabilities or who are struggling with personality problems.

Physical education contributes to the overall educational experiences of an individual, and the physical education teacher is a vital part of the educational team. The goal of each teacher in a school is to help each student to be prepared for life. A physical education teacher uses physical activity to contribute to this goal; a math teacher uses math; and an English teacher uses literature and communication skills. For each, the goal is the same but the context for achieving that goal is different.

PROFESSIONAL RESPONSIBILITIES OF PHYSICAL EDUCATION TEACHERS

Four major responsibilities of physical education teachers are instruction, curriculum development, administration, and collaboration.

Instructional Responsibilities

Physical education teachers must not only devise a physical education curriculum, but they must also instruct students in the setting of the physical education "classroom." Unlike the traditional classroom used by colleagues in other disciplines, the physical education classroom contains no desks, chairs, or lab tables. A physical education instructor's classroom is more likely to be a gymnasium, swimming pool, or playing field. Teaching in several different environments challenges the versatility of physical educators, for it is much different teaching an activity outdoors than it is in the gymnasium, and teaching in the gymnasium is greatly different from the classroom. Competent physical educators are usually well prepared to offer instruction in any of those venues.

To keep abreast of the dynamics of their subject matter, physical education teachers, like their colleagues in other disciplines, remain students themselves. For their own professional development, teachers attend workshops, seminars, and conferences to keep pace with the latest developments in their fields. With childhood obesity nearing epidemic proportions, physical educators might look for professional meetings that will provide them with information for helping obese children combat this condition through a variety of strategies, including diet and exercise. School districts often sponsor in-service programs for teachers to expand their knowledge and grow professionally. In-service programs are generally held on site at one of the schools in the sponsoring district. For physical educators, an authority on adventure education might present a workshop on building confidence and developing trust through the use of low rope elements (obstacles constructed from ropes and other devices one to three feet off the ground that require cooperation and teamwork to traverse).

Some physical education teachers enroll in graduate programs to acquire additional knowledge and bring new ideas and educational experiences to their students. One trend is for individual teachers to develop their own faculty development plan, which is approved by a group of peers. This plan may include graduate courses, but it may also include workshops, attendance at conventions, and/or curriculum writing. The most important issue is that teachers are expected to be learning and improving continuously. A number of states are beginning to require a set number of what is termed "professional development hours" (that is, attending workshops, conferences, and the like) in order to maintain their teaching certification. To encourage professional growth, most school districts reimburse teachers for attending professional meetings and reward them with increases in salary for earning college credits beyond the bachelor's degree.

In addition to participating in standard professional development programs, physical educators must often obtain additional certifications to carry out their instructional responsibilities. If their job description calls for teaching health or driver education, they must seek additional certifications in each of those areas. Depending on licensing requirements that vary from state to state, health certification can require anywhere from twelve to thirty credits, and driver education may take an additional three to twelve credits. Physical educators also need special certifications to teach first aid, cardiopulmonary resuscitation (CPR), swimming, or adventure education. CPR certification must be renewed annually, and the first-aid and lifeguarding or water-safety certifications require renewal at regular intervals. Some states even require a certification for coaches, which means another certification for physical educators who want to coach athletic teams. Conscientious physical educators are dedicated professionals who eagerly seek and maintain additional certifications in the areas in which they want to excel. They are intrinsically motivated to improve and use professional development opportunities to enhance their teaching and, if need be, coaching qualifications.

An important aspect of instruction is the assessment of student progress in physical education. Through observation and performance drills and tests, the instructor evaluates the progress of students. Students can be provided with feedback to help them improve at any activity they undertake. Assessments eventually will be calculated into a grade to inform students, parents, administrators, and others about each student's progress in class. For a physical education teacher who instructs students daily in a traditional seven-period day, the number of students for whom grades must be calculated can range from 150 to 250 pupils. A physical education teacher (usually elementary), who has ten classes a day and only instructs students a couple of times a week might have twice as many grades to calculate.

Curriculum Development

Developing a curriculum is a time-consuming group effort. To develop an effective and sound pre-K to grade 12 curriculum, physical education teachers representing all grade levels become part of a curriculum committee. This committee's first order of business is to design a physical education mission statement for the school district and then determine curricular content to reflect that mission. The curriculum must meet both school district and state physical education content standards. The committee will need to review such materials as the National Physical Education Content Standards developed by the National Association of Sport and Physical Education (NASPE). In building a standard physical education curriculum consisting of movement education, fitness/wellness education, physical performance skills, and lifetime activities, the committee will need to consider students' backgrounds and needs, the community environment, and facilities and equipment available.

The specific types and variety of physical education activities that can be offered are contingent upon space, class size, and number and qualifications of instructors. The imagination and creativity of the instructor can often compensate for large, overcrowded classes in limited space with little equipment. For instance, an ingenious teacher may be able to teach floor hockey to forty children in half of a cafeteria with cardboard hockey sticks and balls made from nylon hose, but the same instructor would not be able to teach swimming without a pool.

School size is another factor. Large schools tend to have two or more physical education teachers, while the smaller ones usually hire only one. In the smaller schools, the lone physical educator is most likely a generalist performing a myriad of duties and teaching all the curricular offerings, which might include dance, fitness activities, team sports, individual and dual sports, martial arts, and the like. In a large school with several physical educators on the faculty, teachers are more apt to be specialists, and one physical educator may teach all dance classes, while another may be responsible for fitness classes.

Administrative Responsibilities

Administrative duties generally escalate for physical educators as they gain more experience and move into supervisory positions with additional responsibilities. A physical educator in a one-person department may handle everything from distributing lockers and issuing padlocks to planning a budget and ordering equipment. In multiperson departments, however, one physical education teacher is appointed department head to run the department and to supervise its other members. Department chairs have multiple responsibilities that involve personnel evaluations, curriculum development, communication with school administrators and district directors of physical education as well as all the routine matters (equipment, facilities maintenance, and so on) necessary to keep a program running. Supervisory responsibilities often involve observing each faculty member as they teach and then offering advice to help each teacher improve. At times, department chairs are asked to make recommendations about a faculty member's reappointment, promotion, tenure, and salary increases.

The physical educator who also coaches often becomes the athletic director responsible for scheduling athletic events and practices, hiring coaches and game officials, arranging transportation, and numerous other duties. At some schools, the chair of physical education also serves as athletic director and, in this dual role, usually has no teaching responsibilities. In some locations two different individuals serve as athletic director and department chair. Depending on the size of the school, they may or may not have teaching duties along with their administrative responsibilities.

Collaboration

Most schools encourage **collaboration** with colleagues in other disciplines. In addressing the needs of the whole child, the school seeks information about all aspects of a pupil's attributes in a learning environment. Through collaboration, a process in which teachers from each discipline (language arts, science, math, and the like) meet periodically to discuss student progress and impediments, teachers identify and discuss problem areas that might inhibit learning as well as successful strategies that enhance learning. It behooves the physical educator to become a part of collaboration teams, in order to provide input from a much different perspective than the classroom teacher can. Collaboration teams are found in middle schools and, to a lesser degree, at high schools where specialists teach in each discipline. At the elementary school level, child-study teams include specialists (school psychologist, speech therapist, reading specialist) along with the classroom teacher. Here, too, the physical educator has much information to offer and should look to share knowledge with other child-study team members.

OTHER PROFESSIONAL RESPONSIBILITIES

Physical education teachers are sometimes expected to coach sport teams, advise cheerleaders, or supervise drill teams. They also organize physical education clubs and intramural activities. The clubs may include such groups as juggling, rope jumping, and general fitness. Physical education teachers are also expected to serve on committees and to attend faculty meetings. Budget problems facing many schools have made it necessary for physical education teachers to develop public relations savvy. As a result, these teachers may need to plan physical education programs similar to music programs, athletic halftime shows, field days, and other activities that focus community attention on the curriculum and the value of physical education. Other responsibilities may include writing articles for newspapers and soliciting media coverage of physical education events. Presentations to home-school organizations and other community and business groups can contribute to community awareness of the importance of fitness and physical education programs in schools. Some ways to publicize physical education and gain recognition for its contributions might be making a report at a faculty meeting, writing an article for a faculty newsletter, and suggesting and organizing a theme week, such as "Healthy Heart Week" or "Fitness Week."

PROFESSIONALISM AND PROFESSIONAL ORGANIZATIONS

Professional organizations are advocates of a particular field because they are composed largely of members who work in that field. Through the membership process, the professional organization brings unity to individuals with similar interests and goals. It brings its members together. The organization holds national and regional conventions, communicates with its members via newsletters, flyers, and mailings, and disseminates information to them through its professional journals. In physical education, the primary national organization is the American Alliance for Health, Physical Education, Recreation and Dance (AAHPERD). Structurally, it consists of six associations representing health, physical education, women's sports, recreation, active lifestyles, and dance. Geographically, it is composed of six districts: eastern, southern, midwest, central, northwest, and southwest. Each state has its own association, which automatically belongs to the district in which it is located. For example, New York belongs to Eastern District Association and Florida belongs to Southern District Association. AAHPERD holds a national convention each year that rotates among four regions. It also publishes several professional journals that disseminate valuable information to its members. The *Journal of Physical Education and Recreation* (*JOPER*) and *Strategies* are most helpful to physical education teachers. AAHPERD also publishes the *American Journal of Health Education* and the *International Electronic Journal of Health Education* for teachers of health and *Research Quarterly for Exercise and Sport* for researchers in the physical education profession.

One effective way for physical educators to keep abreast of the latest developments in their field is to join a professional organization, such as AAHPERD. In fact, it behooves every physical educator to be a member of AAHPERD and the state organization, because significant information about the field flows back and forth between the organization and its members. Through its communication channels, educators disseminate information about new ideas and developments related to the field, debate and discuss controversial issues, and identify and offer solutions to problem areas. The dedicated professional physical educator will hold membership in at least one professional organization.

REASONS FOR TEACHING PHYSICAL EDUCATION

In deciding whether a teaching career is of interest to you, consider both the rewards and challenges of teaching. Some of the rewards of teaching are the joy experienced in helping

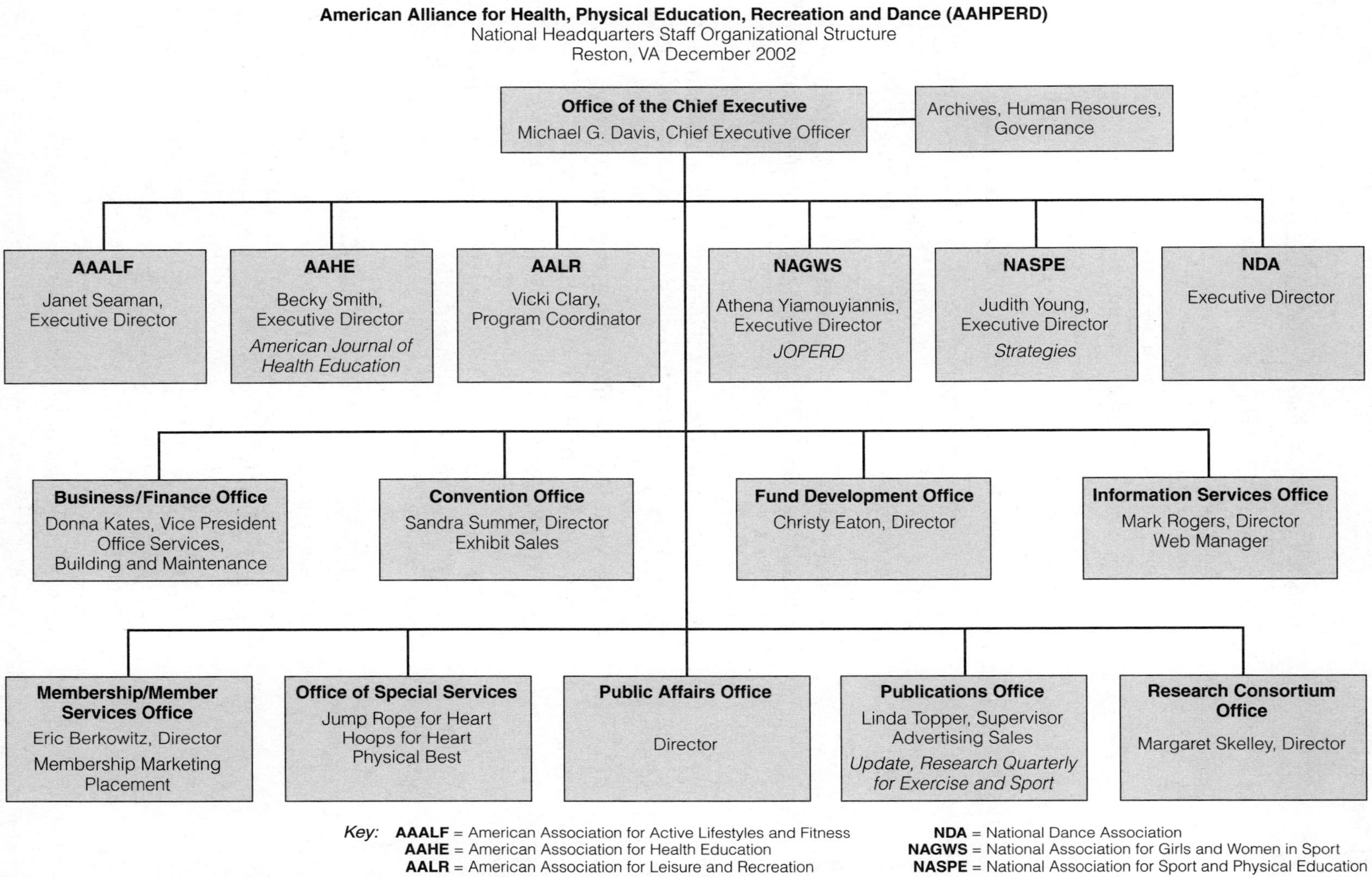

American Alliance for Health, Physical Education, Recreation and Dance (AAHPERD)
National Headquarters Staff Organizational Structure
Reston, VA December 2002

Key: **AAALF** = American Association for Active Lifestyles and Fitness
        AAHE = American Association for Health Education
        AALR = American Association for Leisure and Recreation

NDA = National Dance Association
NAGWS = National Association for Girls and Women in Sport
NASPE = National Association for Sport and Physical Education

Figure 8.1 AAHPERD, initially grounded in physical education, now stretches across four disciplines.

Table 8.1 Reasons to Teach Physical Education

1. The reward of watching students succeed and the joy they experience in doing so
2. The opportunity to work closely with students
3. The opportunity to be physically active during the day
4. The opportunity to watch students grow and mature
5. The opportunity to work with other teachers who share the same interests in student well-being
6. Teaching a wide variety of activities

a child or adult learn: in seeing the "light bulb" come on, seeing a child smile in gratification at something mastered, recognizing a student's improvement in attitude and behavior, and making students feel comfortable in a physical education environment. Teachers say it is gratifying at the end of the school year when students see and feel the benefits of a lifestyle that promotes physical fitness and good health. It is rewarding to gain the respect of students, fellow faculty members, and community residents and to watch students grow and mature.

The rewards of teaching are not monetary, nor does teaching bring one a great deal of prestige. The rewards of teaching are believing that you can make a difference in the lives of students and then actually seeing that happen. Sometimes a thank you is given, but most often the effect a teacher has on a student goes unrecognized. The bottom line is that teachers teach because they love it and they enjoy children.

CHALLENGES TO TEACHING PHYSICAL EDUCATION

One of the most frustrating challenges facing all teachers is apathy. A good teacher is a good motivator and a good observer. But some students dislike physical activity; and when they participate, it is usually grudgingly. The causes of their apathy might lie in being infatuated with video games, having inactive parents who encourage a sedentary lifestyle, or being the subject of ridicule from peers for performing a physical skill poorly. Then, too, a student who is overweight may be uncomfortable participating in physical activity.

Table 8.2 Challenges Facing Physical Education Teachers

1. Apathy—from students and parents
2. Little class time with students
3. Large classes
4. Limited equipment
5. Teaching a wide variety of activities
6. Providing quality programs in difficult financial circumstances
7. Weather causing changes in lesson plans
8. Students with disabilities or poor social skills
9. Defending the need for quality physical education
10. Lack of respect from other teachers and administrators
11. Keeping pace with technology in physical education
12. Motivating students to be active outside of school
13. Loss of teaching areas for school programs
14. Isolation from other teachers
15. The need to be a proper role model for students
16. Grading in physical education
17. Getting to know all students as individuals

Another challenge facing physical education today is making the most of the time available for physical education classes. As states begin to elevate standards in such subjects as mathematics and language arts, principals are dedicating more class time to those subjects. Because there is no interest in increasing the length of the school day or school year, class time for other subjects, like physical education, is decreased. On the elementary level, it is not unusual for a physical education class to meet only once a week for approximately thirty minutes. That means only about thirty-six sessions per year, or eighteen hours of opportunity to develop motor skills and fitness habits. A typical middle school may have physical education every day for fifty minutes for just one semester per year. Some high schools require only one year of physical education. Time constraints make it difficult for physical education teachers to help students improve their motor skills and experience a variety of activities, yet, at the same time, they challenge physical educators to use their ingenuity to provide students with experiences that will facilitate motor skill development within a limited time frame.

The size of physical education classes is a further challenge, especially when classes consist of forty or more students. In some settings, a teacher can offer individual assistance to a student for only one minute of class time. This situation becomes more acute with a shortage of equipment and lack of space, reducing even further the amount of practice time for each student in the class. The challenges for physical education professionals are obvious.

Many of the activities included in a quality physical education program take place most appropriately out of doors. Weather can force a teacher to cancel outside activities, creating the need to have an alternative lesson plan ready on any given day. Another weather-related challenge arises due to changes in conditions throughout the day. For example, early-morning soccer classes may not be appropriate or safe due to the wet ground from the dew and cold temperatures, but in the afternoon the conditions outside for a soccer class may be fine. Insuring that morning classes and afternoon classes receive the same experiences can be difficult.

Students with disabilities often require more individual attention than other students. These students are those with either physical or mental disabilities or both. Federal legislation and mainstreaming have caused the number of special needs students in physical education classes to increase substantially. These students, however, present both a challenge and a unique opportunity for physical educators to help young people in need.

It is not uncommon to find that the value of quality physical education programs is not fully appreciated by administrators and teachers in other disciplines. It is, therefore, in the interests of physical education professionals to inform and enlighten their colleagues of the broad benefits of physical education. These benefits reach far beyond the school yard and the school years.

All teachers are challenged by having to keep pace with the advances in technology. In physical education, there are software programs with superimposed holographic images that depict the correct techniques for performing most sports skills—for example, kicking a soccer ball or pitching a softball. They can be used effectively in lessons involving sports skills. Individual heart-rate monitors are effective in fitness classes as are software packages that calculate caloric intake and energy expenditure. Learning about and implementing new technology requires a great deal of time and effort, but once a teacher masters the useful programs, students are the prime beneficiaries.

One of the most important objectives of physical education is to prepare individuals to be active for a lifetime. In part, this means helping students develop necessary physical skills, but it also means inculcating in them habits of regular physical activity. Physical education teachers reinforce the benefits of regular physical activity; and in doing so, they often initiate attitudinal changes that lead to active lifestyles.

Another challenge that physical educators face is isolation from other teachers. The location of the gymnasium, usually on a corner or one end of the building away from other areas, can contribute to feelings of isolation by reducing opportunities for the physical education teacher to interact with other teachers. Consequently, physical educators have to make an extra effort to communicate and socialize with teachers in other disciplines.

COACHING

As faculties in schools mature and grow older, the number of individuals willing to coach has begun to dwindle. As a result, new teachers, especially those with physical education backgrounds, are often expected to coach. Typically, new physical education teachers begin as an assistant coach in the high school or a head or assistant coach in the middle school. And an ability to coach more than one sport is highly valued. Physical education teachers will find themselves in a stronger position if they have prepared themselves for coaching duties along with teaching. It is not uncommon for elementary school physical education teachers to coach a high school sport. High school coaching positions are not limited to high school teachers only.

To be a successful coach an individual also needs to be a good teacher, able to develop talent from within the school population. Coaches often use the same teaching techniques the physical educator uses; coaching, like teaching, requires dedication, commitment, and self-motivation. Generally, successful coaches are highly organized and competitive. They have thorough knowledge of their sport and manage time well.

OTHER SPORT AND FITNESS SPECIALISTS IN SCHOOLS

A range of sport and fitness specialists may be associated with large schools. These specialists include athletic trainers, aerobic dance teachers, athletic directors, aquatic directors, adapted physical education coordinators, and wellness coordinators. In smaller schools, the roles played by these individuals are often fulfilled by the physical education teacher.

FUTURE OF PHYSICAL EDUCATION FROM PRE-K TO GRADE 12

The changes that have occurred in the United States during the last few years will have an impact on the future of physical education. Student problems are becoming more severe and include discipline problems, disabilities, substance abuse, obesity, a lack of respect for authority, and decreased physical skills. The schools, including the physical education teachers, are expected to do more to prevent and resolve the student problems. The curriculum in physical education is also moving from a sport skills focus to more of a wellness and/or physical fitness approach. Technology, too, will make a big impact on how physical education is taught.

In the future the opportunities for teachers to contribute to bettering the lives of students and, indirectly, parents, will continue to increase. Every time and every place has its own set of problems, but every problem presents an opportunity for a solution. In the future the job of teaching physical education will offer more opportunities to contribute to student and community well-being. Movement toward a wellness-based curriculum will grow stronger, and teachers will be required to use technology to a greater extent. The community will increasingly come to value physical education as physical educators become a recognized resource for parents and others.

In summary, physical educators will be held more accountable for student learning. Implementation of state and national standards means that there will be more opportunity for creative teaching, greater use of technology, and increased need for working with teachers in other disciplines in a partnership to develop the whole child. The need to contribute to character development will mean a curricular shift to adventure education and confidence building, trust formation, and leadership development activities.

ALLIED CAREERS IN FITNESS, SPORT, AND RECREATION

Traditionally, careers in physical education and sport have focused on teaching and coaching in schools, colleges, and universities. Physical education and sports students may discover before, during, or even after their student teaching internship that teaching is not what they really want to do for the rest of their professional career. Some physical education and sports professionals may decide to seek careers in an allied profession that involves fitness, athletic training, sports management, or recreation and leisure. Some may move into an **allied field** after becoming certified in physical education, while others begin to prepare for a career in an allied profession when they matriculate as an undergraduate student. Exciting opportunities exist in many commercial professions, health spas and fitness clubs, community centers, and the corporate world.

The Fitness Industry

Opportunities for a career in fitness education abound in health spas and fitness clubs, corporate fitness centers, private agencies, community institutions, cardiac rehabilitation sites, retirement communities and centers for older adults, and physical and occupational therapy practices. Exercise and fitness specialists, in addition to mastering core physical education requirements—physiology of exercise, biomechanics, and motor learning—need advanced courses in cardiovascular physiology, strength training and conditioning, and neuromuscular physiology. Some even earn a bachelor's degree in exercise science. Whether their degree is in exercise science or physical education, exercise and fitness specialists often enhance their credentials by obtaining certification as an exercise specialist or fitness instructor from a recognized certifying agency. The most reputable for exercise and fitness is the American College of Sports Medicine (ACSM), which has two certification tracks—Clinical and Health/Fitness. For those interested in strength training, the National Strength and Conditioning Association (NSCA) offers certification in that area.

Exercise and fitness specialists can work in health spas and fitness clubs where they prescribe and supervise exercise programs of club members. They might also conduct group exercise programs. Some opt to set up their own personal training practice in which they work individually with a number of clients. Others seek positions in a corporate fitness setting where they perform essentially the same functions for business executives. Most specialists at corporate fitness sites hold a master's degree, though advanced degrees are not necessary for employment at all corporate locations. Other agencies and institutions where exercise and fitness specialists find work are YM-YWCAs, YM-YWHAs, Boys and Girls Clubs, and community centers that offer exercise programs.

With special training in cardiovascular physiology and exercise stress testing, exercise and fitness specialists can work in cardiac rehabilitation centers, which are usually located in hospitals or clinics. In this setting, exercise specialists assist and monitor cardiac patients with their post-operative rehabilitative exercise programs. A master's degree is advantageous in obtaining work in cardiac rehabilitation.

As the older adult population in the United States continues to increase, there is a crucial need to help older adults remain independent for as long as possible. Exercise specialists and fitness instructors, with their background in physiology of exercise, can help immeasurably. They must have had gerontology courses dealing with the exercise limitations caused by the aging process, and they must know how to prescribe appropriate exercises that are compatible with the strength, cardiovascular, flexibility, and functional capacities of the older adults with whom they are working. Exercise specialists who are qualified to work with older adults can perform a valuable service for the older adult population and for society in general. They may find employment in retirement communities, older-adult apartment complexes and assisted living quarters, community centers and nutrition sites where older adults congregate, and nursing homes.

Some physical therapists and occupational therapists will hire exercise specialists to assist them in their patients' rehabilitation process. While the physical or occupational therapist uses various modalities (heat, ultrasound, electrical stimulation) as well as manual manipulation in the therapeutic process, the exercise specialist, under the direction of the physical or occupational therapist, will monitor and guide the patient through a program of rehabilitative exercises. Graduates with a background in exercise physiology or athletic training are normally found in this environment.

Athletic Training

Initially emerging out of the physical education curriculum as a minor or concentration, athletic training, over the past two decades, has carved out its own identity as a separate academic major on numerous campuses. In fact, the National Athletic Trainers' Association (NATA) and the Council for the Accreditation of Allied Health Education Programs (CAAHEP) are now requiring all undergraduate curriculum programs that prepare students for careers in athletic training to convert to a major in athletic training by fall 2005. In the past, students would major in physical education and take a concentration of courses, twenty-one to thirty credits, in athletic training, ranging from preventing and caring for athletic injuries to internships as trainers with high school and college athletic teams. Upon completing the athletic training curriculum, a student would then take the NATA examination to become a certified athletic trainer. Generally, a certified trainer works with athletic teams on the high school, college, or professional level. The trainer's primary duties are to devise conditioning and training programs for athletes in order to prevent injuries and to help athletes recover when injuries do occur. Most trainers work on the high school level, where increasing numbers of school districts are requiring dual certification in athletic training and teaching. Athletic trainers may also work in sports medicine clinics, physical and occupational therapy clinics, or private practices.

Sports Management

The field of sports management prepares one for managerial, marketing, and administrative positions in some sporting venue, usually on the professional or collegiate level, although opportunities for sports management graduates are opening up in the corporate world. Students prepare for this allied career by taking courses in business and sport courses involving the social sciences and humanities. Graduates of sports management programs who get the glamour positions with professional sports teams usually begin their careers as administrative assistants responsible for ticket sales, special promotions, community relations, and a variety of other tasks related to the marketing of the club or team—as do those who start their careers assisting an athletic director at a college or university. If new graduates start in minor league baseball or basketball, they may play a more prominent role. Some graduates may find work assisting with or managing a sporting or multipurpose facility, such as an arena, stadium, swimming pool, golf course, tennis club, health spa, or fitness center. In the corporate world, the sports management graduate might be involved in the sale or marketing of sporting goods, fitness equipment, sports memorabilia, team souvenirs, and sports advertising. As with the situation in exercise science, the sports management graduate with an advanced degree will generally fare better in this competitive marketplace.

Recreation and Leisure Pursuits

Graduates with a background in recreation can find employment at amusement parks, theme parks, and state, municipal and national parks. They may also work as recreation directors in towns and cities, community centers (YM-YWCAs and Boys and Girls Clubs, among others), private agencies (nursing homes, senior centers), and retirement communities. Recreation specialists might also be found running summer camps of all types or managing golf courses, tennis courts, and racquetball clubs. At most colleges and universities, recreation is a separate major; in some, recreation is a concentration or minor embedded within the physical education curriculum. The recreation curriculum often combines managerial courses with outdoor education (botany and zoology as well as outdoor activities, such as swimming, canoeing, and rock climbing), arts and crafts, and active and quiet group activities. A career in recreation offers a wide array of options.

Other Allied Careers in Sport

Among other allied professions are sports communication—which offers opportunities as journalists, broadcasters, or technicians—and sports officiating. A career in sports communication requires special skills—in writing for journalists and in speaking for broadcasters (who also need effective voice resonance). Technicians need special skills with television, video, and computer equipment for televising or broadcasting sporting events. To pursue a career as a sports journalist, sports broadcaster, or sports technician, it is advisable to major in communication.

Physical educators and athletic coaches generally pursue sports officiating for supplemental income rather than as a career. Those who seek a career as an official will need special training and preparation beyond what is offered in physical education programs. Major and minor league baseball umpires attend and graduate from umpiring schools. Basketball officials can work their way up from high school to college competition, but making it to the professional game is quite difficult and highly competitive. Football officiating, at all levels, is a part-time, weekend position that provides supplemental income.

CHOOSING A CAREER

Choosing a career in physical education and sport involves a decision-making process that considers desire, character, personal strengths, interest, preparation, on-the-job experiences, and goals. Explore your selected career opportunities by gathering information (refer to Web sites), evaluating data, and continuously reevaluating your decisions.

At this time in your life, you may not know whether to pursue a career in teaching or in an allied field. Now is the time for you to explore your interest in the field of physical education and the growing number of opportunities that are available.

Today in our physical activity, fitness, and sports-oriented world, a background in physical education/sport can provide you with numerous avenues toward selecting a fulfilling and rewarding career that can match your personal interests. But how do you know which career is best for you? First, be versatile; consider more than one specific area. Second, be mindful that it is natural to change your opinion about a career several times during your college years and perhaps several more times during your working years. The important message at this point in your life is to keep your mind open to all options and gather as much information as possible about each career path. Then, through the evaluation process, you will be able to make an informed decision.

On the Web

www.pe4life.org
Good for promoting physical education; contains research, resources, and latest news.

http://www.walktoschool-usa.org
This site includes information about Walk to School Day and how to plan your own event.

http://www.brentwood.k12.mo.us/Middle%20School/ Mr%20I's%20PE%20Page/mripe.htm
A physical education teacher's Web site; includes a wealth of information about his physical education program as well as links to other important sites.

http://askeric.org/cgi-bin/lessons.cgi/physical_education
Site contains lesson plans on games, motor skills, skill related lessons, gymnastics, outdoor education, and team sports.

http://www.stan-co.k12.ca.us/calpe
California Physical Education Resources Web site contains resources for curricular matters, fitness, funding, current topics, and other Web sites.

http://www.ccsso.org/intasc.html
This site discusses what INTASC is and provides links to the ten INTASC Standards and state education agencies.

http://www.nbpts.org
The site provides information about national standards and how to get national board certification.

http://www.nationjob.com
Career and job Web site; helpful in locating jobs.

http://humankinetics.com
Human Kinetics site provides descriptions of different physical activity careers, job search strategies, and professional organizations.

http://outwardbound.org
Outward Bound Web site provides information on adventure activities.

http://onlinesports.com/sportstrust/
Site contains back issues of *Sports News You Can Use* with information on sports business and careers, sports promotion, event marketing, and retailing.

http://www.bls.gov/oco
The Occupational Handbook Web site provides information about different occupations, working conditions, job outlook, earnings, and training.

Key Terms

allied fields The fields of health, recreation, dance, athletic training, and sports management that share some purposes, programs, and professional activities with physical education and sport (page 187).

certification A statement or document indicating the fulfillment of requirements that grants one permission to practice or carry out occupational duties in a specific field (page 170).

collaboration Process in which teachers from each discipline work together to identify and discuss problems that inhibit learning. Collaboration can also occur between the school and two or more entities in the community (page 178).

profession An occupation requiring specialized education and training; a profession usually has a set of standards for entry and a certification or licensing process (page 170).

wellness Physical, mental, emotional, nutritional, and spiritual factors that lead to healthy lifestyle behaviors (page 173).

Multiple Choice Questions

1. The organization that has developed national standards for beginning physical education teachers, which numerous states have adopted is
   a. NASPE
   b. NBPTS
   c. INTASC
   d. NCAA
   e. NAPEHE

2. Physical education teachers observe students interacting with one another through physical activity, which provides the educational community with another dimension for assessing the students'
   a. mathematical skills
   b. reading skills
   c. writing skills

    d. social skills

    e. vocational skills

3. The purpose of a "faculty development plan" is to help physical education teachers

    a. stay current with latest developments

    b. change careers

    c. unseat the principal

    d. reduce paperwork

    e. get out of the gym

4. The process in which teachers from various disciplines meet to discuss student progress and impediments is known as

    a. integration

    b. disintegration

    c. accentuation

    d. configuration

    e. collaboration

5. The professional organization that represents the physical education profession on the national level is

    a. NCAA

    b. USOC

    c. AAHPERD

    d. AAKPE

    e. ACLU

6. One of the greatest challenges facing physical education teachers today is

    a. apathy of students

    b. overzealous students

    c. bountiful budgets

    d. small class sizes

    e. abundance of space

7. Which *one* of the following is *not* true about the roles and responsibilities of physical education teachers?

    a. changed little over the past several years

    b. often includes coaching

    c. includes promotion and marketing physical education

    d. involves curriculum writing

    e. may have administrative duties

8. Expectations for the future of physical education include all *but one* of the following. Which one is not included?

    a. increased use of technology

    b. more adventure-type activities

    c. greater concern for wellness

    d. unlimited budgets

    e. increased emphasis on fitness

9. Physical educators enter the teaching profession because they

    a. will become wealthy

    b. love children

    c. will become famous

    d. will advance socially

    e. will enter politics

10. Choice of career is generally influenced by

    a. interests and goals

    b. academic preparation

    c. character and personal strengths

    d. experiences

    e. all of the above

Critical Thinking Questions

1. If we believe, as our tradition tells us, that physical education is predicated on physical activity and wellness, then the physical educator is in a vital position to promote this concept. Should physical education teachers be models of fitness, wellness, and sound health practices, or can they advocate these values and lifestyle without personally living them? Explain your answer with a logical argument.

2. Numerous physical education teachers also coach athletic teams. Oftentimes coaching duties and responsibilities conflict with the goals of physical education by reducing the amount of time a physical education teacher can put into planning and preparing lessons for physical education. Construct a sound argument that supports physical educators undertaking high school coaching assignments.

3. Evaluation and grading are sometimes controversial issues in physical education. How should physical education students be evaluated? Should they be graded on scores made on physical performance and fitness tests, improvement, class participation, attendance, attitude, or a combination of any or all of these variables? Develop your answer with a sound, logical argument for whatever mechanism(s) you would use for evaluation.

4. Some administrators and teachers in other disciplines do not fully understand the nature of physical education and its role in the schools. How would you go about enlightening a school principal and colleagues in other disciplines about the benefits of physical education and what exactly would you say?

5. Making a career choice and selecting an undergraduate major can be difficult decision for some students who have just graduated from high school. What advice would you give to a high school graduate who participated in athletics in high school and is leaning toward majoring in physical education?

References

Centers for Disease Control and Prevention. *Guidelines for School and Community Programs: Promoting Lifelong Physical Activity.* U.S. Department of Health and Human Services, 1997.

Delpy, L. A. "Career Opportunities in Sport: Women on the Mark." *Journal for Physical Education, Recreation, and Dance, 69,* no. 7 (1998): 17–21.

Harrison, J. M., Blakemore, C. L., and Buck, M. M. *Instructional Strategies for Secondary School Physical Education,* 5th ed. Dubuque, Iowa: McGraw-Hill, 2001.

International Life Sciences Institute. *Improving Children's Health through Physical Activity: A New Opportunity, A Survey Of Parents and Children about Physical Activity Patterns.* Washington, D.C.: International Life Sciences Institute, 1997.

Lumpkin, A. *Physical Education and Sport: A Contemporary Introduction,* 5th ed. Boston, Mass.: McGraw-Hill, 2002.

National Association for Sport and Physical Education. *Moving into the Future: National Standards for Physical Education.* St. Louis: Mosby, 1995.

National Association for Sport and Physical Education. *Shape of the Nation Report: Status of Physical Education in the USA.* Reston, Va.: American Alliance for Health, Physical Education, Recreation and Dance, 2001

National Collegiate Athletic Association. *NCAA Gender Equity Study: Summary of Results 1997.* Overland Park, Kans.: National Collegiate Athletic Association, 1998.

Pestolisi, R. A., and Baucher, C. *Introduction to Physical Education: A Contemporary Careers Approach,* 2nd ed. Glenview, Ill.: Scott/Foresman, 1990.

Siedentop, D. *Introduction to Physical Education, Fitness, and Sport,* 5th ed. New York: McGraw-Hill, 2003.

Tillman, K. G., Voltmer, E. F., Esslinger, A. A., and McCue, B. F. *The Administration of Physical Education, Sport and Leisure Programs.* Boston, Mass.: Allyn and Bacon, 1996.

United States Olympic Committee. *97/98 Factbook.* Colorado Springs, Colo: United States Olympic Committee, 1997

Women's Sports Foundation. *Gender Equity Report Card.* East Meadow, N.Y.: Women's Sports Foundation, 1997.

Women's Sports Foundation. *Women's Sports Facts.* East Meadow, N.Y.: Women's Sports Foundation, 1997

Women's Sports Foundation. *Women's Sports Foundation Insider.* East Meadow, N.Y.: Women's Sports Foundation, 1997.

Wuest, D. A., and Bucher, C. A. *Foundations of Physical Education, Exercise Science, and Sport,* 14th ed. Boston, Mass.: McGraw-Hill, 2002.

9

ISSUES AND OPPORTUNITIES IN PHYSICAL EDUCATION

Chapter Objectives

After reading this chapter, the student will be able to

- Define hypokinetic disease and indicate remedies through physical education

- Identify major advantages and disadvantages of physical education programs based on fitness, skill development, or competitive games

- Discuss strategies for promoting equality in issues involving gender, disabilities, age, ethnicity, and sexual orientation

- Explain the nature and benefits of adventure education and interdisciplinary units

This chapter will introduce issues and describe opportunities currently important in physical education. We won't be able to settle these issues, but perhaps an awareness of them will lead to further inquiries on your part and constructive discussions and debates. Some of the issues are controversial and others are less so, but all of them affect education in general and physical education in particular. We will look at hypokinetic disease and the intervention of physical education; curricular matters and controversies; equality issues involving gender, disabilities, age, ethnicity, and sexual orientation; and current trends and future opportunities.

HYPOKINETIC DISEASE AND THE INTERVENTION OF PHYSICAL EDUCATION

The American Heart Association has recently classified **hypokinetic disease,** or too little physical activity, as a controllable risk factor for heart disease. The incidence of hypokinetic disease has been increasing in the United States since the midpoint of the twentieth century. The image of the United States as a nation of doers built upon rugged individualism, robust vigor, and relentless energy seems to represent the past, not the present, as we enter the twenty-first century. This unnerving predicament is due largely to advancements in technology and changes in public policies and popular practices.

Over the past fifty years, Americans' devotion to the automobile has discouraged walking and bicycling, their infatuation with television and computer games has kept them indoors and diminished their interest in physical activity, their apathy at the voting booth has enabled states and school districts to reduce physical education requirements, and their abdication of civic responsibilities has allowed communities to minimize the new construction and maintenance of parks, playgrounds, and public recreation facilities.

All of those developments and practices have contributed to declining levels of physical activity among Americans of all ages. In fact, the Centers for Disease Control and Prevention (CDC) have reported that only 25 percent of adults

Adults

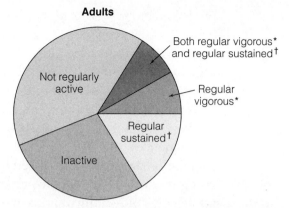

* Regular Vigorous—20 minutes 3 times per week of vigorous intensity
† Regular Sustained—30 minutes 5 times per week of any intensity

Source: CDC 1992 Behavioral Risk Factor Survey

Figure 9.1 Growing inactivity among American adults. Barely 35 percent participate in regular physical activity each week.

perform activities that were considered moderately active on five or more days each week,[1] while the Surgeon General has discovered that 40 percent of all adults refrain from participating in any leisure-time physical activity at all.[2] Less than one-third of all adults engage in the recommended amounts of physical activity (thirty minutes) at least three times each week.

For children and adolescents, the figures are equally bleak. Nearly half of the United States' youth in the twelve- to twenty-one-year-old age bracket and more than one-third of high school students do not participate in vigorous physical activity on a regular basis. Among youth, activity seems to decline as age increases. Ninth-graders (72 percent) partake in more vigorous physical activity than do high school seniors (55 percent). Less than 25 percent of children get twenty minutes or more of vigorous physical activity each day. At all grade levels, boys receive more vigorous physical activity than girls do. Among all age groups inactivity or hypokinetic disease and poor diet cause an estimated 300,000 deaths a year.[3]

Hypokinetic disease, moreover, is directly related to overweight and obesity, an epidemic that is sweeping the United States as we begin the twenty-first century. The recently published *Surgeon General's Call to Action to Prevent and Decrease Overweight and Obesity, 2001,* revealed that 61 percent of American adults were either overweight or obese. Over the past two decades, the prevalence of obesity and overweight in children between the ages of six and eleven has increased from 7 to 13 percent; and in adolescents aged twelve to nineteen, it has nearly tripled to 14 percent. The consequences of the United States' overweight and obese population are seen in increased health problems and rising medical costs. When compared with children and adolescents of healthy weights, overweight children and adolescents have higher cholesterol levels and blood pressures, two risk factors associated with heart disease, and a greater incidence of type 2 diabetes, heretofore considered an adult disease. More alarming is the prospect that overweight adolescents have a 70 percent chance of bringing that condition into adulthood. The health risk factors for overweight and obese adults are heart disease, hypertension, stroke, type 2 diabetes, breathing problems, arthritis, certain types of cancers, and such psychological disorders as depression. The Surgeon General's report reveals increased risk of premature death associated with overweight and obesity, and CDC researchers estimate a potential savings of $76.6 billion in medical costs if all inactive Americans became physically active.[4]

Physical education is a perfect antidote to hypokinetic disease, and its timely intervention can play a huge role in improving the health and physical condition of our nation. Intervention at this juncture gives physical education professionals a great opportunity to grasp the reins of leadership in this campaign against overweight and obesity. As advocates and models of physical activity, physical education teachers must cultivate in school-age children positive attitudes toward exercise and physical activity. Through enticing programs and exciting experiences, teachers can motivate children to remain physically active throughout their entire lifetimes. Overweight and obesity saddle their victims with another burden—social discrimination—which devastates one's self-esteem and self-confidence. Here, too, physical educators are in a pivotal position to help. They can

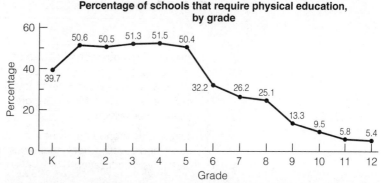

Figure 9.2 The CDC's recently conducted School Health Policies and Programs Study (SHHPS) shows required physical education decreasing from grades 5 to 12.

build confidence in children of all shapes and sizes by elevating their activity levels through challenging program offerings that allow for success.

In order to stem the tide of overweight and obesity, the profession of physical education, from AAHPERD and other national bodies down to regional and state organizations, must convince government officials at all levels of the physical activity needs of Americans in all age groups. Physical educators must gain the support of elected officials, at least tacitly if not fiscally, to sustain existing programs and to create new ones where necessary. Although most states and school districts require physical education at the elementary-, middle- and high school levels, the *School Health Policies and Programs Study (SHHPS) 2000* revealed that only 8 percent of the elementary schools, 6 percent of the middle/junior high schools, and 6 percent of the high schools require daily physical education for each grade level throughout the entire year. Furthermore, the *SHHPS* survey found that the percentage of schools requiring physical education in each grade declined from 50 percent in grades 1–5 to 25 percent in grade 8 and to 5 percent in grade 12.[5]

These findings challenge the physical education goals of *Healthy People 2010,* which calls for the United States to increase daily physical education in public and private schools, to increase the proportion of adolescents who participate in daily physical education, and to increase the

Table 9.1 Healthy People 2010 Physical Activity Objectives

OBJECTIVE	BASELINE	TARGET
Increase the proportion of adolescents who engage in vigorous physical activity that promotes cardiovascular fitness 3 or more days per week for 20 or more minutes per session	65 percent	85 percent
Increase the proportion of the nation's public and private schools that require daily physical education	middle/ jr. high 17%; senior high 2%	middle/ jr. high 25%; senior high 5%
Increase the proportion of adolescents who participate in daily physical education	29 percent	50 percent
Increase the proportion of adolescents who spend at least 50 percent of school physical education class time being physically active	38 percent	50 percent

proportion of adolescents who are physically active during at least 50 percent of their physical education class time.[6] Physical educators and their professional organizations can use these documents and data effectively to promote physical education in their school districts and communities. They can also make sound arguments to civic officials to make facilities for physical activities available to all age groups—facilities ranging from ball fields and gymnasiums for youth sports programs to walking paths and recreational venues for older adults.

While hypokinetic disease, or physical inactivity, is one of the leading causes of overweight and obesity, unhealthy dietary patterns, genetics, and lifestyle also play significant roles. In addition to promoting increased physical activity, physical educators and health educators, along with other school officials and parents, can encourage youth to develop sound eating habits. Dietary guidelines for healthy eating include reducing fat and caloric intake, drinking more water and fewer sugar-flavored beverages, and replacing high-calorie high-sugar snacks with five servings of fruits and vegetables each day.

CURRICULAR MATTERS AND CONTROVERSIES

Physical education curricula are expanding beyond traditional team and individual/dual sports approaches. In this chapter we turn our attention to new concepts and activities: fitness versus skill development, competitive games, and wellness/lifestyle classes.

Fitness versus Skill Development

Whether the physical education curriculum should focus on skill development or fitness has been a topic of considerable discussion and concern. Because public school physical education constantly faces the threat of a reduction in class time or, worse yet, elimination of programs, a growing number of physical educators believe that physical fitness should be the focus of their curriculum. These educators argue that teaching youth about health-related fitness components—cardiorespiratory endurance, strength, muscular endurance, flexibility, and body composition—will be of greater value to pupils over their entire life span than learning the skills to engage in basketball, volleyball, badminton, tennis, golf, and other sports. Fitness advocates maintain that learning how to improve fitness and then to sustain it at appropriate levels is more beneficial to a person's health than mastering a variety of sports skills. Others counter the fitness argument with the supposition that sports and performance skills enable individuals to participate in recreational and leisure time activities throughout their lives. Too much emphasis on developing fitness turns students off, contributing to a negative attitude toward exercise and eventually causing them to withdraw from physical activity.

There is, however, a middle ground in this debate of fitness versus skill development because there is room in the physical education curriculum to accommodate both. Buck and McManama conducted a study to determine whether performance skills and physical fitness could be developed simultaneously. The investigators randomly assigned students to two volleyball classes. One class was taught the game in a traditional manner with the focus on skill development. The

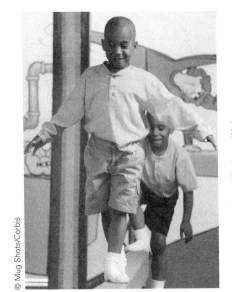

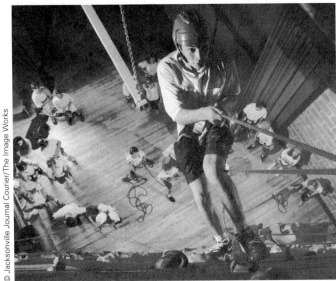

Physical education programs balance fitness training with physical performance and skill development.

other class was induced to increase the amount of movement expected of each student using the performance skills of volleyball. Post-test results revealed that the level of skill development was the same in both classes, but the class that participated in extra movement made significant improvements in cardiorespiratory endurance and flexibility. The findings of this study indicate that both performance skills and physical fitness can be improved concurrently.[7]

Competitive Games

Traditionally, physical education classes have had a competitive focus. This begins early in the school years with relay races and other games in which a score is kept. It continues as sport skills are taught and the focus of some programs turns to playing games. In recent years physical educators have begun to question the value of competition. Some believe that too much competition may be harmful to youth, particularly those who have poor physical performance skills. In **zero-sum competition,** in which there is one winner and one loser, 50 percent of the participants experience failure. For some students, repeated failure lowers their self-esteem and damages their self-confidence. Some physical educators and psychologists argue that students experience plenty of situations in which success is difficult to attain, so physical education classes should provide opportunities for all students to experience success. The counterargument holds that our highly competitive society dictates the need to expose children early to competition so they become adept at handling success and failure in daily living situations.

A number of competitive games (such as king of the ring) are designed to eliminate participants as the activity proceeds. This type of game reduces rather than increases physical activity in a physical education class. Physical educators should strive to teach activities that maximize participation in the brief time period they have with their pupils. Because most states and school districts do not require daily physical education for all students, physical educators have to be prudent and innovative in selecting activities that allow for maximum participation throughout the entire class period. Granted, maximizing participation requires more time, effort, and creativity in planning lessons, but it also provides physical educators with an opportunity to demonstrate their desire to give their pupils sound educational experiences.

Another component of the competition model is **non-zero-sum competition,** in which contestants try to improve upon their previous time, distance, or score in a run, throw, or other activity—or they give their best effort in trying to reach or eclipse a predetermined standard in some physical performance event. Physical educators often use non-zero-sum competitive activities to teach important lessons involving success and failure.

Some competitive games, by their very nature, are inappropriate for physical education classes because of their potential to cause injuries. In an age when violence has been increasing in the schools, games such as dodgeball, killer ball, and murder ball, in which pupils are the target of a thrown object, have no place in the physical education curriculum. Skills such as dodging can be learned through participation in other agility drills and tag games.

Wellness/Lifestyle Classes

Many high schools and a few middle schools are offering physical education or health classes with a wellness lifestyle theme. In some schools these classes are elective, and in others they are required. The classes teach students about all the dimensions of wellness—physical, emotional, intellectual, social, and spiritual. The students complete projects designed to facilitate the adoption of healthy lifestyles. These classes are much more than fitness, physical conditioning, or weight training classes that are available as electives in many high schools. While weight training and physical conditioning may be a part of a wellness program, students also learn how to develop their own exercise programs and adopt appropriate nutrition practices. Topics related to emotional, social, intellectual, and spiritual dimensions of wellness are also included.

EQUALITY ISSUES INVOLVING GENDER, DISABILITIES, AGE, ETHNICITY, AND SEXUAL ORIENTATION

In physical education, as in the larger arena of sport, discrimination of all types, whether wittingly or not, did exist and probably still does in some circles. With federal legislation and declarations, protests and movements by affected minority groups, and litigation and court orders, some progress toward equality for disaffected groups has been made. Because of **Title IX,** more women and girls participate in sport than ever before. Several pieces of federal legislation in the last quarter century have given individuals with disabilities the same educational opportunities as those without disabilities. The political clout of older adults, the fastest-growing segment of the United States' population, has brought them some relief and increased benefits. Although prejudice against ethnic and geographical groups is far from eradicated, the civil rights movement triggered legislation that has opened doors previously closed to African Americans, Latinos, and other ethnic minorities. Gay and lesbian protests and demonstrations have heightened aware-

Table 9.2 Female High School (NFSHSA) and Collegiate (NCAA) Participation

		1971–72	2000–01	PERCENT INCREASES
High School Varsity Athletes	Female	294,015	2,784,154	847
	Male	3.666,917	3.921,089	6.9
Collegiate Varsity Athletes	Male	170,384	208,866	35.1
	Female	29,977	150,916	411

Source: National Coalition of Women and Girls in Education, "Title IX Athletics Policies; Issues, and Data for Education Decision Makers," A Report from the National Coalition for Women and Girls in Education, August 27, 2002. Washington, D.C.: American Association of University Women

ness of their plight. The quest for equality by each oppressed group has affected physical education.

Title IX of the Education Amendments Act of 1972

Growing out of the civil rights crusade and feminist movement of the 1960s came Title IX of the Education Amendments Act of 1972. This landmark piece of legislation required institutions to provide equal opportunity and equal funding for programs or activities receiving federal financial assistance. Although its greatest impact was felt in the realm of athletics, where female participation on sports teams at all levels (high school, college, Olympics) has increased enormously,[8] Title IX was largely responsible for coeducational classes in physical education. Prior to 1972 most physical education classes from middle/junior high school upward were separated according to gender. Early on, physical education's leadership, seizing the opportunity to promote gender equity within their profession, endorsed Title IX. Some rank-and-file members, in the spirit of providing girls and women with equal access to quality physical education experiences, facilities, and equipment, integrated their classes quickly, while others, who had known only gender-segregated classes for decades, took longer to adopt the coeducational model. Failure to comply with Title IX can result in the loss of federal aid and the payment of monetary damages to anyone who a court of law finds has been harmed due to unequal educational opportunities.

Students with Disabilities

Students with disabilities bear a double burden. The disability not only places them at a disadvantage with the general student population in executing physical performance skills, but it also tends to separate them from their classmates. In order to give pupils with disabilities as many natural experiences as possible, educators have attempted to include all students together in classes as much as possible. At one time, students with disabilities were placed in special schools or in their own classroom with limited exposure to other students. Now educators make every effort to place these students in the **least restrictive environment.** As a consequence, students with disabilities participate in regular physical education classes whenever possible.

In 1990 the **Individuals with Disabilities Education Act (IDEA)** (PL 101-476) was passed. This law updated the 1975 Education for All Handicapped Children Act (PL 94-142). The law stated that all students with disabilities are entitled to an education in the least restrictive environment without any additional expense to the parents or guardians. All students with an identified disability are required to have an **individualized education program (IEP)** developed for them. The IEP identifies the student's present level of performance and provides guidance for the development of an appropriate physical education curriculum for each student with a disability.

An earlier law designed to provide equal opportunity for individuals with disabilities that has affected physical education is Section 504 of the Rehabilitation Act of 1973 (PL 93-112). This law requires all students to have an equal opportunity to participate in all programs provided by the school. Students must have access to all buildings and facilities and transportation. Appropriate equipment is also

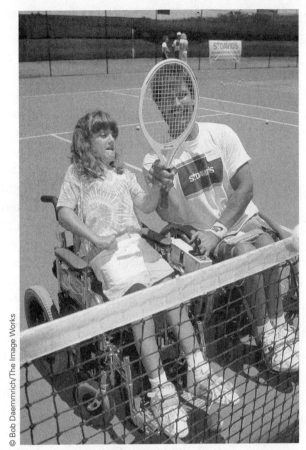

© Bob Daemmrich/The Image Works

Physical education is inclusive and attempts to accommodate students with disabilities or impediments.

needed to enable students with disabilities to participate in physical education classes.

Physical education teachers, therefore, must have sufficient background in providing equal educational opportunities for students with disabilities. Physical education majors, who have the opportunity to complete a minor or certification in adapted physical education, are knowledgeable about integrating disabled students in their physical education classes. An additional benefit accrues to physical educators who receive in-depth training in adapted physical education. They are in greater demand as more and more schools are enrolling more students with disabilities.

Older Adults

The United States' older adult population, currently at 35 million, is expected to double by 2030, with a 50 percent rise coming by 2020. These demographic projections present the physical education profession with additional opportunities and challenges. Older adults need physical activity in order to remain independent and to carry out tasks of daily living (such as personal hygiene, dressing, eating). Physical educators, with their background in exercise and motor behavior, have rudimentary knowledge to help older adults remain active. Granted, physical educators are prepared essentially to work with children from pre-K to grade 12, but much of what they have learned about exercise and physical activity can be applied to the older adult population as long as they recognize and understand the physical limitations of older adults. With some additional courses in gerontology, physiology of exercise, motor behavior, psychology of aging, and death and dying, physical educators would be well prepared to work with the older adult population.

National certifications for conducting exercise and activity programs for older adults are under development. Physical educators, with the preparation outlined above, should seek such certification when it becomes available. Until that time, physical education majors, interested in working with older adults, should consider a minor or concentration in exercise gerontology, if one is available at their institution. If none is available, they might consider building their own cluster of courses in exercise gerontology in consultation with an academic adviser who is knowledgeable about exercise physiology and gerontology.

Ethnic and Geographical Diversity

Just as the United States' population continues to grow older, it is also becoming more ethnically diverse. In order to keep pace with these changing demographic patterns, teacher preparation programs must build into their curricula experiences that give prospective teachers sufficient exposure to ethnically diverse groups. Most physical education programs have field work experiences in urban, suburban, and rural settings that cut across a variety of ethnic lines. These experiences are designed to give prospective teachers a better understanding of the culture of students from diverse backgrounds. The aim, of course, is to prepare teachers who will be effective with all groups under difficult conditions. And in the broader perspective of American society, teacher preparation programs that emphasize **diversity** foster ethnic harmony in a nation that has struggled to overcome discriminatory practices in its pursuit for equality.

Sexual Orientation

Long a taboo topic in American culture, sexual orientation has been put on the table and openly discussed in recent decades. For centuries, gays, lesbians, bisexuals, and transsexuals have borne the brunt of harassment and discrimination. As a result of antidiscrimination and sexual harassment legislation, many gays and lesbians feel comfortable publicly announcing their sexual orientation. In physical education, professional organizations often include workshops and seminars about sexual orientation at their national and regional conventions in the interest of abating discrimination and encouraging empathy.

CURRENT TRENDS AND FUTURE OPPORTUNITIES

In focusing on current trends and future opportunities, we will discuss such topics as adventure education, interdisciplinary involvement, and the potential of technology.

Adventure Education

Adventure education includes backpacking, orienteering, camping, canoeing, and some risk-taking activities involving ropes courses and climbing apparatus. These activities contribute to the development of muscular strength and endurance and cardiorespiratory endurance. Adventure activities stimulate the psychomotor domain and positively influence the affective domain, which deals with habits and attitudes that reinforce participation and enhance well-being. Self-confidence and self-efficacy increase as a result

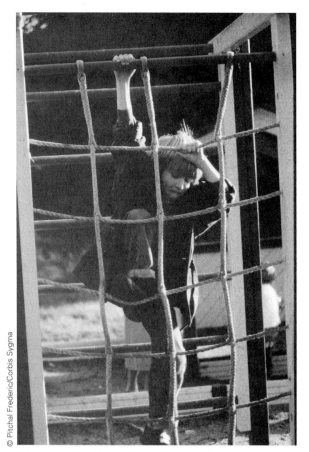

© Pitchal Frederic/Corbis Sygma

Adventure education builds confidence and trust among students.

of completing ropes courses and other risk-taking activities. Other benefits accrued are team building, cooperation, and respect for the decisions others make.

Recognizing the value of adventure education, a number of schools are building climbing walls, installing ropes courses, and incorporating camping, orienteering, and other outdoor activities into the curriculum. Other schools are working within their communities to develop outdoor adventure areas in cooperation with the community and neighboring schools. Established teachers are urged (and expected) to become certified in the instruction and safety required for these types of activities. New teachers coming into physical education will be expected to enter the job market with certification to conduct adventure education activities.

Interdisciplinary Involvement

Educators have discovered the educational benefits of connecting different subjects to one another in an **interdisciplinary units** format. Because mathematics, science, and English are usually taught as separate subjects, isolated from one another, students are not aware of the many fascinating interrelationships among disciplines. Middle schools especially have been sensitive to this concern and have initiated a team-teaching approach to provide interdisciplinary experiences. The team consists of one teacher from each subject area, plus specialty teachers in physical education, music, art, and other areas. This approach allows teachers to develop and teach in an interdisciplinary environment and helps students make connections that add relevancy to what they are learning.

Physical educators can also initiate interdisciplinary units. Several units are available commercially or teachers may design one or more of their own. A physical education interdisciplinary unit should use skills such as throwing, catching, climbing, running, jumping, and striking to represent an event or activity. For example, in the Heart Adventure students throw a ball through hoops hung from the ceiling, run, and pull themselves along a rope while sitting on a scooter and holding a ball in their laps. Students simulate blood cells traveling around the heart and then through the rest of the body. As the students actively experience the path the blood takes through the heart, they learn the names of each section of the heart along with the valves regulating blood flow between chambers.[9] The teacher can also illustrate what happens when a person's lifestyle contributes to such diseases as arteriosclerosis.

Other subject areas, too, can include activities and discussions related to the heart. In mathematics classes, for example, students can determine the number of heartbeats during sleep, or they can practice using decimals to determine upper and lower limits of target heart-rate zones that are used for cardiorespiratory exercise programs. Social studies classes can study the incidence of heart diseases in various parts of the world and the effects different lifestyles have on heart disease. In English classes students can write about their experiences in the heart adventure activity or can prepare research reports on the heart. Music classes can discuss heartbeat rhythm or perform songs that have "heart" in their titles.

Interdisciplinary activities add interest, opportunities for critical thinking and problem solving, and experiential learning. Moreover, interdisciplinary activities often—and importantly—make learning fun.

The Potential of Technology

By the latter decades of the twentieth century, technological developments and devices had already made substantial inroads in the physical education learning environment. Video cameras and recorders provide instant feedback to prospective teachers as they perform their demonstration lessons in pedagogy courses and fieldwork experiences. The computer, ubiquitous in education, has brought software packages to the gymnasium to facilitate teaching and learning sports skills. Some sophisticated packages, not readily affordable for most school districts at this time, even provide holographic images of successful performers that can be superimposed over a pupil's freshly recorded movement patterns in order to compare correct sports skills techniques with the novice's. In due time, however, production costs of this equipment and technology will come down to a level that most school districts can afford.

Interactive television (ITV) classrooms enable classes at two or more different sites (schools) to be hooked up with one another. This technology has worked well for social studies, English, foreign language, and other classroom-based courses. It enables smaller schools to receive course offerings not available at their location. In the preparation of physical education teachers, ITV can be used in pedagogy courses to broaden students' experiences. For instance, a physical education lesson at an off-campus site might be beamed back to an undergraduate pedagogy class where students can analyze class organization, teaching styles,

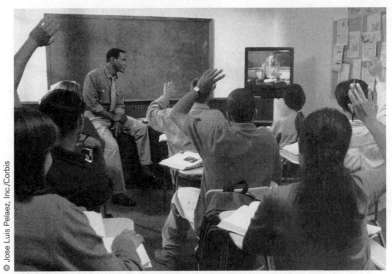

© Jose Luis Pelaez, Inc./Corbis

Learning is a two-way process as these students in an interactive classroom are learning through two environments.

class management, discipline, and time devoted to physical activity. Then over time, other lessons from urban, suburban, and rural sites might be transmitted back to the college for comparative analyses of teaching in these three venues. Outdoor-indoor pedagogical connections for lesson evaluation in these two different environments may also prove to be valuable.

In recent years the use of heart-rate monitors in physical education classes has enabled students to observe and record accurate heart-rate measurements before, during, and after cardiorespiratory endurance training. Software packages can process and analyze recordings for an entire class. With this technology, teachers and pupils not only get a more accurate picture of the heart's response to exercise, but also save valuable class time previously spent on measuring pulse rate manually and then recording the measurement.

Then, too, technological improvements in safety devices (eye guards, padding, and the like) and sports, fitness, and games equipment (ranging from floor hockey sticks to tennis racquets) have enhanced safety and facilitated learning.

Creative Scheduling

Physical education, unlike classroom subjects, does not always fit into standard class-time periods. On the elementary level, it is not unusual for a class to meet just twice a week for about twenty-five to thirty minutes. This amount of time is not sufficient for the development of performance levels to match the national and state outcomes established for each grade level. Part of the promotion of an elementary physical education program is to propose alternative scheduling that will increase opportunities for elementary students to participate in physical education for longer periods each week. Another means of accomplishing this goal is to provide classroom teachers with curricular ideas to be used on days when the students do not come to physical education class.

At the secondary level, **block scheduling** is beginning to command more attention. Two basic types of block schedules exist—Block 4 and Block 8. In each case, the students have a four-period day rather than a seven- or eight-period day. Under this scenario, each class period is approximately ninety minutes long. Teachers still have one preparation period each day that goes for ninety rather than fifty minutes. In the Block 4 plan, students take four classes in one block. Each class meets everyday for four and one-half weeks. The Block 8 system allows students to take as many as eight classes in one block. The student attends the same classes on alternate days, four classes on day one and four more on day two. This typically means the school has an A-day and a B-day (often school colors are used to designate one day from the other). Block 8 is more popular than the Block 4 system. Students keep this schedule for the entire school year, though elective classes might meet for half a year.

Teachers prefer the extra preparation time provided by block schedules. Physical education teachers welcome longer class periods for imparting information and teaching students to master the physical education curriculum. Classroom teachers, however, have found the ninety-minute class period a challenge to their teaching techniques, which may have to change in order to hold student interest throughout the entire class. While the extended period is a boon to physical education teachers, they must use the time effectively with creative lessons to induce learning. Visionary teacher education programs will prepare future teachers to use block schedules effectively.

Marketing and Fund-Raising

In this era of fiscal prudence and limited resources brought about by taxpayer resistance and state budget deficits, school districts are forced to reduce costs in order to function within their budgetary allotment. School districts cut costs by removing personnel, reducing student services, or canceling equipment orders.

In order to maintain current staff, services, and programs, schools have begun public relations and marketing campaigns to raise sufficient funding to keep their programs going. Some schools have attracted corporate sponsors either to renovate an old gymnasium or to build a new one. In return for their financial contributions, the corporation name and logo will appear on a building or facility.

The expense necessary to keep abreast with technology is often beyond the financial capacity of school districts. To deal with this dilemma, more school districts are seeking gifts from business and industry and grants from public and private foundations. Computers, fitness, nutrition, and performance-skill software packages, video cameras and recorders, and other technologies are needed the most. The schools and school districts that promote themselves within and outside the community, undertake serious fund-raising efforts, and reach out to parents, politicians, and community leaders will secure sufficient monies to carry out their educational mission.

On the Web

http//www.cdc.gov/
Official Web site of the Centers for Disease Control and Prevention. Contains a wealth of information about health and physical activity items.

http://www.high5adventure.org
The official Web site of High 5 Adventure Learning Center, an organization that provides information and materials for adventure education activities.

http://www.ropesonline.org
Ropes Online is devoted to the development and marketing of
ropes/challenge course programs.

http://www.dol.gov/oasam/regs/statutes/titleix.htm
Text of Title IX legislation, Education Amendments of 1972.

http://bailiwick.lib.uiowa.edu/ge/
An excellent site for securing information on all aspects of issues of gender equity in sports. It includes recent cases and Title IX resources and
statistics.

http://www.cdc.gov/nccdphp/sgr/sgr.htm
Information about the Surgeon General's Report on Physical Activity
and Health as well as the Executive Summary.

Key Terms

adventure education A curriculum area that includes outdoor activities,
such as backpacking, orienteering, camping, canoeing, and rock climbing, as well as controlled risk-taking activities on low and high ropes
courses to develop trust, confidence, and cooperation (page 213).

block scheduling Method of scheduling in which, classes meet for longer
periods of times (usually twice the length or a traditional period or ninety
minutes); there are fewer periods each day and usually fewer days of instruction. In block scheduling, the instruction is more concentrated (page 218).

diversity Heterogeneous mix of religion, ethnicity, gender, and sexual
orientation in groups of people in various environments; for our purposes, in the educational setting (page 213).

hypokinetic disease Lack of or too little activity; a controllable risk factor of coronary heart disease (page 200).

Individuals with Disabilities Education Act (IDEA) A law passed in
1990 that stated that all students with disabilities are entitled to an education in the least restrictive environment (page 210).

individualized education program (IEP) Program that outlines the educational placements appropriate for a student with an identified disability; also identifies present levels of performance and goals for the
future (page 210).

interdisciplinary unit A unit of instruction in which several curriculum
areas are taught together, either in one curricular area or in cooperation
with several curriculum areas (page 215).

interactive television (ITV) Service that enables instruction to occur in
two or more settings simultaneously through technology of two-way
video and audio communication (page 216).

least restrictive environment Term for requirement that all students be placed in the setting that will result in the best opportunity for success and educational progress. Placements range from a special adapted physical education classroom to inclusion in the regular physical education classroom with no adaptations (page 210).

non-zero-sum competition Situation in which participants work to meet a predetermined standard or improve their own previous best performance; contrasted with traditional competition that has winners and losers (page 207).

Title IX Part of the Education Amendments Act of 1972, the law requires every educational program receiving federal assistance to provide equal opportunities for males and females (page 208).

zero-sum competition Traditional competitive situation in which the outcome leads to one winner and one loser (page 206).

Multiple Choice Questions

1. The lack of or too little physical activity is a condition known as
   a. hyperkinetic disease
   b. hypokinetic disease
   c. hyperactive disease
   d. hypodermic disease
   e. hyperthermia disease

2. The percentage of American youth (ages twelve to twenty-one) who do not participate in vigorous physical activity on a regular basis is nearly
   a. 25 percent
   b. 33 percent
   c. 50 percent
   d. 66 percent
   e. 75 percent

3. In 2001 the Surgeon General revealed that the percentage of overweight and obese adults in the United States has risen to
   a. 31 percent
   b. 41 percent
   c. 51 percent
   d. 61 percent
   e. 71 percent

4. Outdoor educational experiences combined with some risk-taking activities on ropes and climbing apparatus is known as
   a. cooperative games
   b. fitness games

    c. adventure education

    d. interdisciplinary learning

    e. movement education

5. The law that requires equal educational opportunities for females and males, including coeducational physical education classes is

    a. IDEA

    b. Section 504

    c. Title IX

    d. PL 94-142

    e. SHHPS

6. IEP is an abbreviation for

    a. Individualized Education Project Plan

    b. Individualized Education Program

    c. Institutional Education Package

    d. Instructional Education

    e. Individual Equity Plan

7. One of the most recent creative scheduling innovations is

    a. module scheduling

    b. traditional scheduling

    c. core scheduling

    d. block scheduling

    e. cluster scheduling

8. IDEA (PL 101-476) entitles all students to an education in the

    a. least responsible environment

    b. least restrictive environment

    c. least representative environment

    d. most responsible environment

    e. most restrictive environment

9. Combining learning experiences from two or more subject areas simultaneously is known as

    a. cooperative games

    b. fitness games

    c. adventure education

    d. interdisciplinary learning

    e. movement education

10. Two or more classes at different sites can be taught simultaneously with two-way technology known as

    a. ITV classroom

    b. WHO classroom

    c. SHHPS classroom

    d. IEP classroom

    e. IDEA classroom

Critical Thinking Questions

1. The Surgeon General and the Centers for Disease Control and Prevention (CDC) have provided overwhelming evidence of a childhood obesity epidemic in the United States. What are the causes of this epidemic, and what can you do as a physical educator to reduce the level of childhood obesity?

2. In designing and developing their curricula, physical educators have wrestled with the notion of emphasizing fitness over performance skill development, and there is good reason given the incidence of childhood obesity. As a prospective physical education teacher who will one day be involved in designing curricula, what would you emphasize and why?

3. Competition has long been a component of physical education programs and classes. As you prepare for a career as a physical education teacher and possibly an athletic coach, too, how will you use competitive games in your physical education program?

4. Since the advent of Title IX in 1972, coeducational classes have become increasingly commonplace in our nation's schools. Reflect upon your experiences, perhaps as a student in coed physical education classes, by identifying the strengths and shortcomings of this situation, and then explain what you would do to make the learning environment as attractive and as beneficial as you can for both boys and girls.

5. Interdisciplinary units consist of integrating one or more classroom subjects (math, English, social studies, and the like) with physical education. Take one classroom subject and indicate how you would combine some of its major concepts with physical education.

References

Acosta, R. V., and Carpenter, L. J. "Courtside: Seven Questions about Title IX." *Strategies,* 11, no. 1 (1997): 31–33.

Benham Deal, T., and Deal, L. O. "Heart to Heart: Using Heart Rate Telemetry to Meet Physical Education Outcomes." *The Journal of Physical Education, Recreation & Dance,* 66, no. 3 (1995): 30–35.

Blakemore, C. L., and Rogers, J. K. "Learn How Middle School Students Think." *Strategies,* 8, no. 5 (1995): 11–14.

Block, M. E. "Americans with Disabilities Act: Its Impact on Youth Sports." *The Journal of Physical Education, Recreation & Dance,* 66, no. 1 (1995): 28–32.

Block, M. E. "Modify Instruction: Include All Students." *Strategies,* 9, no. 4 (1996): 9–12.

Block, M. E., and Etz, K. "The Pocket Reference—A Tool for Fostering Inclusion." *The Journal of Physical Education, Recreation and Dance,* 66, no. 3 (1995): 47–51.

Block, M. E., Lieberman, L. J., and Connor-Kuntz, F. "Authentic Assessment in Adapted Physical Education." *The Journal of Physical Education, Recreation & Dance,* 69, no. 3 (1998): 48–55.

Boyce, B. A., and Markos, N. "Advocacy—Links to the Community." *Strategies,* 9, no. 2 (1995): 22–25.

Boyce, B. A., and Nelson, T. D. "The Underground Railroad: A Multi-cultural, Interdisciplinary Project." *Strategies,* 8, no. 2 (1994): 20–23.

Buck, M. M. "Interdisciplinary Approach to Teaching: K–12 Physical Education." *Journal of Interdisciplinary Research in Physical Education,* 1, no. 1 (1996): 7–14.

Buck, M. M., and Kirkpatrick, B. "Find Funds for Wellness Assessment Equipment." *Strategies,* 8, no. 5 (1995): 5–9.

Buck, M. M., and McManama, J. *Improving Skill & Fitness Concurrently: Can It Be Done?* Poster session presented at the 38th World Congress of the International Council for Health, Physical Education, Recreation, Sport and Dance, Gainesville, Florida, July 1995.

Centers for Disease Control and Prevention. *Guidelines for School and Community Programs: Promoting Lifelong Physical Activity.* U.S. Department of Health and Human Services, 1997.

Claxton, D. B., and Bryant, J. G., Jr. "Block Scheduling: What Does It Mean for Physical Education?" *The Journal of Physical Education, Recreation & Dance,* 66, no. 3 (1996): 48–50.

Colven, A. V., and Walker, P. J. "Map Out Success." *Strategies,* 9, no. 7 (1996): 26–29.

Copeland, B. W. *Funding Sources in Physical Education, Exercise, and Sport Science.* Morgantown, W. Va.: Fitness Information Technology, 1995.

Corbin, C. B., and Pangrazi, R. P. *Physical Activity for Children: A Statement of Guidelines.* Reston, Va.: National Association for Sport and Physical Education, 1998.

Crouch, S., editor. *Speaking of Fitness . . . Commentaries on Youth Physical Fitness.* Reston, Va.: American Alliance for Health, Physical Education, Recreation and Dance, 1996.

Crouch, S., Meredith, M., Cain, L., and Corbin, C. B. *You Stay Active.* Reston, Va., and Dallas, Tex.: American Alliance for Health, Physical Education, Recreation and Dance and Cooper Institute for Aerobics Research, 1995.

Davis, M. G. "Promoting Our Profession: The Best of Times . . . the Worst of Times." *The Journal of Physical Education, Recreation & Dance,* 67, no. 1 (1996): 48–51.

Fried, G. "Courtside: ADA Q&A." *Strategies,* 10, no. 5 (1997): 23–25.

Friesen, R., and Bender, P. "Internet Sites for Physical Educators." *Strategies,* 11, no. 1 (1997): 34–36.

Fullerton, J., and Madjeski, H. E. "Group Initiative Strategies for Addressing Social Issues." *The Journal of Physical Education, Recreation & Dance,* 67, no. 5 (1996): 52–54.

Gass, M. A., and Williamson, J. "Accreditation for Adventure Programs." *The Journal of Physical Education, Recreation & Dance,* 66, no. 1(1995): 22–27.

Grosse, S. J. "Send Your Students Out to Cruise." *Strategies,* 11, no. 1 (1997): 18–20, 29.

Harrison, J. M., Blakemore, C. L., and Buck, M. M. *Instructional Strategies for Secondary School Physical Education,* 5th ed. Dubuque, Iowa: McGraw-Hill.

Harvard Center for Cancer Prevention. *Harvard Center for Cancer Prevention Report Calls for Increased Physical Activity to Reduce Cancer Risk.* 1997. http://bw/971210/harvard_cancer_preve_1.html

Henderson, K. A. "Marketing Recreation and Physical Activity Programs for Females." *The Journal of Physical Education, Recreation & Dance,* 66, no. 6 (1995): 53–57.

Henkel, S. A. "Monitoring Competition for Success." *The Journal of Physical Education, Recreation & Dance,* 68, no. 2 (1997): 21–28.

Houston-Wilson, C., Lieberman, L., Horton, M., and Kasser, S. "Peer Tutoring: A Plan for Instructing Students of All Abilities." *The Journal of Physical Education, Recreation & Dance,* 68, no. 6 (1997): 39–44.

Hudgins, J. L., and O'Connor, M. J. "Let The Surgeon General Help Promote Physical Education." *The Journal of Physical Education, Recreation & Dance,* 68, no. 8 (1997): 61–64.

International Life Sciences Institute. *Improving Children's Health through Physical Activity: A New Opportunity, A Survey Of Parents and Children about Physical Activity Patterns.* Washington, D.C.: International Life Sciences Institute, 1997.

Jambor, E. A., and Weekes, E. M. "Videotape Feedback: Make It More Effective." *The Journal of Physical Education, Recreation & Dance,* 66, no. 2 (1995): 48–50.

Kahan, D., and McKnight, R. "Personal Responsibility in the Gymnasium." *Strategies,* 11, no. 3 (1998): 13–17.

Kasser, S. L., Collier, D., and Solava, D. G. "Sport Skills for Students with Disabilities: A Collaborative Effort." *The Journal of Physical Education, Recreation & Dance,* 68, 1 (1997): 50–53, 56.

Kirkpatrick, B., and Buck, M. M. "Heart Adventures Challenge Course: A Lifestyle Education Activity." *The Journal of Physical Education, Recreation & Dance,* 66, no. 2 (1995): 17–24.

Kleinman, I. "Grading: A Powerful Teaching Tool." *The Journal of Physical Education, Recreation & Dance,* 68, no. 5 (1997): 29–32.

Mills, B. "Opening the Gymnasium to the World Wide Web." *The Journal of Physical Education, Recreation & Dance,* 68, no. 8 (1997): 17–19.

Mills, B. D., and Mitchell, C. A. *Jumpstart with Web Links: A Guidebook for Sport Education and Activities.* Englewood, Colo.: Morton, 1997.

Mittelstaedt, R. D. "Climbing Walls Are on the Rise: Risk Management and Vertical Adventures." *The Journal of Physical Education, Recreation & Dance,* 67, no. 7 (1996): 31–33, 36.

Mittelstaedt, R. "Indoor Climbing Walls: The Sport of the Nineties." *The Journal of Physical Education, Recreation & Dance,* 68, no. 9 (1997): 26–29.

Mohnsen, B., Chestnutt, C. B., and Burke, D. "Multimedia Projects." *Strategies,* 11, no. 1 (1997) 10–13.

Mohnsen, B., and Schiemer, S. "Handheld Technology: Practical Application of the Newton Messagepad." *Strategies,* 10, no. 5 (1997): 12–14.

Murata, N. M., and Hodge, S. R. "Training Support Personnel for Inclusive Physical Education." *The Journal of Physical Education, Recreation & Dance,* 68, no. 9 (1997): 21–25.

National Association for Sport and Physical Education. *Appropriate Practices for High School Physical Education.* Reston, Va.: NASPE, 1998.

National Association for Sport and Physical Education. *Moving into the Future: National Standards for Physical Education.* Reston, Va.: NASPE, 1995.

National Association for Sport and Physical Education. *Outcomes of Quality Physical Education Programs.* Reston, Va.: NASPE, 1992.

National Association for Sport and Physical Education. *Physical Education Program Improvement and Self-Study Guide: Middle School.* Reston, Va.: NASPE, 1998.

National Association for Sport and Physical Education. *Physical Education Program Improvement and Self-Study Guide: High School.* Reston, Va.: NASPE, 1998.

National Association for Sport and Physical Education. *Shape of the Nation Report: A Survey of State Physical Education Requirements.* Reston, Va.: NASPE, 1998.

National Association for Sport and Physical Education. *Sport and Physical Education Advocacy Kit*. Reston, Va.: NASPE, 1994.

Pangrazi, R. P., and Corbin, C. B. *Teaching Strategies for Improving Youth Fitness*, 2d ed. Reston, Va.: American Alliance for Health, Physical Education, Recreation and Dance.

Pate, R. R., and Hohn, R. C., editors. *Health and Fitness through Physical Education*. Champaign, Ill: Human Kinetics, 1994..

Placek, J. H., and O'Sullivan, M. "The Many Faces of Integrated Physical Education." *The Journal of Physical Education, Recreation & Dance*, 67, no. 1 (1997): 20–24.

Rauschenbach, J. "Tying It All Together: Integrating Physical Education and Other Subject Areas." *The Journal of Physical Education, Recreation & Dance*, 67, no. 2 (1996): 49–51.

Smith, T. K., and Cestaro, N. "Making Physical Education Indispensable: A 10-Point Action Plan." *The Journal of Physical Education, Recreation & Dance*, 67, no. 5 (1996): 59–61.

Spickelmier, D., Sharpe, T., Deibler, C., Golden, C., and Krueger, B. "Use Positive Discipline for Middle School Students." *Strategies*, 8, no. 8 (1995): 5–8.

Staffo, D. F. "Show Off Your Program." *Strategies*, 10, no. 5 (1997): 19–22.

Stanton, K., and Colvin, A. V. "The Physical Educator's Role in Inclusion." *Strategies*, 9, no. 4 (1996): 13–15.

Stier, W. F., Jr. *Fundraising for Sport And Recreation: Step-By-Step Plans for 70 Successful Events*. Champaign, Ill.: Human Kinetics, 1994.

Stier, W. F., Jr. *More Fantastic Fundraisers for Sport And Recreation: 70 Step-By-Step Plans*. Champaign, Ill.: Human Kinetics, 1997.

Strand, B., and Mathesius, P. "Physical Education with a Heartbeat: Part II." *The Journal of Physical Education, Recreation & Dance*, 66, no. 9 (1995): 64–68.

Strand, B., and Reeder, S. "Increasing Physical Activity through Fitness Integration." *The Journal of Physical Education, Recreation & Dance*, 66, no. 3 (1996): 41–46.

U.S. Department of Health and Human Services. *Physical Activity and Health: A Report of the Surgeon General—Executive Summary*. Pittsburgh, Penn.: USDHHS, 1996.

Van Oteghen, S., and Mahood, R. "Reading and Physical Activity: A Natural Connection." *Strategies*, 9, no. 2 (1995): 26–29.

Watters, R. "Navigating from the Classroom to the Outdoors: Teaching Map and Compass. *The Journal of Physical Education, Recreation & Dance*, 67, no. 5 (1996): 55–56.

White, E. "Make Archery a Sport for the Visually Impaired." *Strategies,* 8, no. 8 (1995): 12–14.

Williams, N. F. "The Physical Education Hall of Shame. Part III: Inappropriate Teaching Practices." *The Journal of Physical Education, Recreation & Dance,* 67, no. 8 (1996): 45–48.

Worrell, V., and Napper-Owen, G. "Combine Fitness and Skills. *Strategies,* 8, no. 8 (1995): 9–11.

Notes

1. National Center for Chronic Disease Prevention and Health Promotion, "Nutrition & Physical Activity." 2002, Oct 17. http//www.cdc.gov/nccdphp/dnpa/physicalactivity.htm.

2. U.S. Department of Health and Human Services, *Physical Activity and Health: A Report of the Surgeon General* (Atlanta: U.S. Department of Health and Human Services, Centers for Disease Control and Prevention, National Center for Chronic Disease Prevention and Health Promotion, 1996), p. 4.

3. *The Surgeon General's Call to Action to Prevent and Decrease Overweight and Obesity.* Office of Disease Prevention and Health Promotion; Centers for Disease Control and Prevention, National Institutes of Health. Rockville, Md.: U.S. Dept of Health and Human Services, Public Health Service, Office of the Surgeon General, Washington, D.C., 2001; National Association for Sport and Physical Education, "Shape of Our Nation's Children, Highlights from Recent Studies." 2002, Oct. 17. http://www.aahperd.org/naspe/template.cfm?template=shapeNation.html.; CDC's Guidelines for School and Community Programs, Promoting Lifelong Physical Activity, An Overview. Centers for Disease Control and Prevention, National Institutes of Health, Rockville, Md.: U.S. Dept of Health and Human Services, July 2000. http://www.cdc.gov/nccdphp/dash/physact.htm

4. *The Surgeon General's Call to Action to Prevent and Decrease Overweight and Obesity.* Office of Disease Prevention and Health Promotion; Centers for Disease Control and Prevention, National Institutes of Health, Rockville, Md.: U.S. Dept of Health and Human Services, Public Health Service, Office of the Surgeon General, Washington, D.C., 2001; National Center for Chronic Disease Prevention and Health Promotion, "Lower Direct Medical Costs Associated with Physical Activity." 2002, Oct 17. http//www.cdc.gov/nccdphp/dnpa/press/archive.lower_cost.htm

5. Charlene R. Burgeson et al., "Physical Education and Activity: Results from the School Health Policies and Programs Study 2000," *Journal of School Health,* 71, no. 7 (September 2001): 279–93.

6. U.S. Dept. of Health and Human Services, *Healthy People 2010, With Understanding and Improving Health and Objectives for Improving Health*, 2d ed. Washington, D.C.: U.S. Government Printing Office, 2000.

7. M. M. Buck and J. McManama, "Improving Skill & Fitness Concurrently: Can It Be Done?" Poster session presented at the 38th World Congress of the International Council for Health, Physical Education, Recreation, Sport and Dance, Gainesville, Fla., July 1995.

8. From 1972 when Title IX was instituted until 2001, female high school varsity athletes increased by 847 percent (from 294,015 to 2,784,154) and female collegiate varsity athletes increased by 411 percent (from 170,384 to 208,866). National Coalition for Women and Girls in Education, "Title IX Athletics Policies, Issues and Data for Decision Makers," August 27, 2002. While the percentage of female athletes has jumped dramatically since the inception of Title IX, the percentage of female coaches has not kept pace. Since 1972, the percentage of females coaching female teams has dropped from 90 per cent to 48 percent.

9. B. Kirkpatrick and M. M. Buck, "Heart Adventures Challenge Course: A Lifestyle of Education Activity," *Journal of Physical Education, Recreation & Dance*, 66, no. 2 (February 1995): 17–24.

10

THE FUTURE OF PHYSICAL EDUCATION

Chapter Objectives

After reading this chapter, the student will be able to

- Identify and discuss trends in physical education

- Discuss healthy lifestyles and the prevention of disease. Identify the food groups and servings listed in the Food Guide Pyramid.

- Discuss how technological advances will influence physical education

- Identify and discuss current trends in physical activity programs

- Describe the future direction of physical education

TRENDS IN PHYSICAL EDUCATION

It's the twenty-first century, a new millennium, and there will be even more changes in the directions physical education takes than there were in the last century. How will these changes affect you, your career, and society? No one knows, but we can make predictions about the future based on current trends in the physical education profession. Among the most important trends are a new emphasis on healthy lifestyles and the prevention of disease, changing demographics, and changes in physical education (reflected in programs in schools and colleges, physical activity and fitness programs, technology, and physical education and service learning).

Looking at these trends, we can project future possibilities. As you read about these, consider the implications that these possibilities will have on the future of physical education and how they may affect your future as a physical education professional.

HEALTHY LIFESTYLES AND THE PREVENTION OF DISEASE

There is compelling evidence that lifestyle is clearly associated with most of today's health problems in the United States. Higher risk of disease results from lifestyle decisions and conditions such as physical inactivity; a poor diet (high fat, low-fiber, and minimal fruits and vegetables); weight gain; consumption of alcohol; smoking; and stress. For much of the twentieth century, the American health care system focused on treatment of disease, and prevention was not significantly addressed until the end of the century. According to World Health Organization (WHO) figures, the United States spends more per capita ($3,724 per year) on health care than any other country in the world, yet the health care system ranks only thirty-seventh in the world (see Figure 10.1).

Japan spends one-half of what the United States does per person on health care, and yet the Japanese outlive U.S. residents by an average of five years. The United States also fails to provide good health care for its entire population.

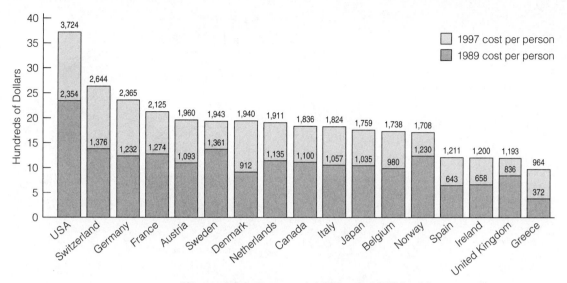

Figure 10.1 Estimated 1989 and 1997 health-care costs per person for selected countries.

Furthermore, forty-four million residents do not have health insurance.

By the time the twenty-first century opened, the American health care system placed primary emphasis on the prevention of disease, a shift from its earlier focus on treatment of disease. Three landmark documents reflect this new focus. First, in 1979, *Healthy People: The U.S. Surgeon General's Report on Health Promotion and Disease Prevention* represented the U.S. government's launch of a plan to establish broad national goals that would promote wellness among all Americans. Those goals were converted into specific health objectives a year later, with a precise list of measurable goals to be attained by 1990. Some of the goals were met, and others were not. The Healthy People 2000 National Health Objectives consisted of a set of goals aimed at taking Americans into the twenty-first century with a higher level of health and wellness. Again some of these goals were met, while others were not, partly because the goals were perceived as unreachable, there was a lack of national financial support, and there was no clear plan for achieving the goals. The goals were again revised with the intent of helping improve

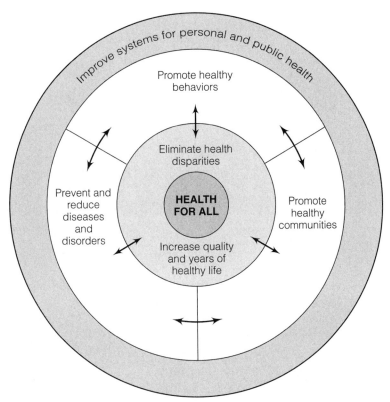

Figure 10.2 National health objectives 2010: Healthy people in healthy communities.

the health of all Americans. Among other goals, the 2010 objectives emphasized increased quality of life during the years of healthy life and sought to eliminate health disparities among all groups of people (see Figure 10.2).

The objectives address three important points:

1. *Personal responsibility.* Individuals need to become ever more health-conscious. Responsible and informed behaviors are the keys to good health.

2. *Health benefits for all people.* Lower socioeconomic conditions and poor health are often interrelated. Extending the benefits of good health to all people is crucial to the health of the nation.

3. *Health promotion and disease prevention.* A shift from treatment to preventive techniques will drastically cut health

care costs and help all Americans achieve a better quality of life.

Figure 10.3 summarizes key 2010 health objectives.

Second, in 1996, the *Surgeon General's Report on Physical Activity and Health* challenged U.S. citizens to improve health through physical activity.

Third, *Dietary Guidelines for Americans, 2000* promotes nutritional guidelines intended for healthy children (two years and older) and adults of any age. These guidelines—based on the available scientific research on nutrition and health and current dietary habits—can potentially reduce the risk of developing certain chronic diseases. The committee issued three goals that include ten guidelines. These goals have been defined as the ABCs for health. Refer to On the Web for additional information concerning the *Dietary Guidelines for Americans, 2000.*

Aim for Fitness

- Aim for a healthy weight.   - Be physically active each day.

Build a Healthy Base

- Let the **Food Guide Pyramid** guide your food choices (see Figure 10.4 on page 238).

- Choose a variety of grains daily, especially whole grains.

- Choose a variety of fruits and vegetables daily.

- Keep food safe to eat.

Choose sensibly

- Choose a diet that is low in saturated fat and cholesterol and moderate in total fat.

- Choose beverages and foods to moderate your intake of sugars.

- Choose and prepare foods with less salt.

- If you drink alcoholic beverages, do so in moderation.

Three factors that do the most for health, longevity, quality of life and the prevention of disease are proper nutrition, a sound exercise program, and quitting (or never starting) smoking. In the future, responsibility for enhancing a healthy lifestyle to prevent disease and making appropriate changes

Figure 10.3 Selected health objectives for 2010.

Mental Health and Mental Illness
- Reduce the suicide rate.
- Reduce the proportion of homeless adults who have serious mental illness.
- Increase the number of states, including the District of Columbia, and territories with an operational plan that addresses mental health crisis interventions, ongoing screening, and treatment services for elderly persons.

Maternal and Child Health
- Reduce fetal and infant deaths.
- Reduce maternal illness and complications due to pregnancy.
- Increase the proportion of pregnant women who receive early and adequate prenatal care.
- Increase the proportion of mothers who breast-feed their babies.

Family Planning
- Increase the proportion of pregnancies that are intended.
- Increase the proportion of females at risk of unintended pregnancy (and their partners) who use contraception.
- Increase the proportion of adolescents who have never engaged in sexual intercourse.
- Reduce the proportion of married couples whose ability to conceive or maintain a pregnancy is impaired.

Injury and Violence Prevention
- Reduce maltreatment and maltreatment fatalities of children.
- Reduce the rate of physical assault by current or former intimate partners.
- Reduce the annual rate of rape or attempted rape.

- Reduce deaths caused by motor vehicle crashes.
- Increase use of safety belts.
- Increase functioning residential smoke alarms.

HIV
- Reduce the incidence of acquired immune deficiency syndrome (AIDS) among adolescents and adults.
- Increase the proportion of sexually active people who use condoms.
- Increase the number of people testing positive for the human immuno deficiency virus (HIV) who know their serostatus.
- Reduce deaths from HIV infection.
- Reduce new cases of perinatally acquired HIV infection.

Sexually Transmitted Diseases
- Reduce the proportion of adolescents and young adults with *Chlamydia trachomatis* infections.
- Reduce gonorrhea.
- Eliminate sustained domestic transmission of primary and secondary syphilis.
- Reduce the proportion of persons with human papillomavirus infection.
- Reduce the proportion of females who have ever required treatment for pelvic inflammatory disease.

Immunization and Infectious Diseases
- Reduce or eliminate indigenous cases of vaccine-preventable diseases.
- Reduce hepatitis A; reduce hepatitis C.
- Reduce Lyme disease.
- Reduce tuberculosis.
- Reduce the number of antiobiotics prescribed for the sole diagnosis of the common cold.

will rest more with the individual. Physical educators will continue to provide knowledge and skills to others by designing individualized exercise programs, promoting lifetime activities, and teaching a variety of stress management techniques.

Childhood Obesity and Diabetes

Obesity in children and adolescents is generally caused by lack of physical activity, unhealthy eating patterns, or a

Figure 10.3 (continued)

Cancer
- Reduce the overall cancer death rate.
- Reduce the lung cancer death rate.
- Reduce the breast cancer death rate.
- Reduce the prostate cancer death rate.

Diabetes
- Prevent diabetes.
- Increase the proportion of persons with diabetes who receive formal diabetic instruction.
- Reduce death from cardiovascular disease in persons with diabetes.
- Increase the proportion of adults with diabetes who self-monitor their blood glucose at least once daily.

Arthritis, Osteoarthritis, and Chronic Back Conditions
- Reduce the proportion of adults with chronic joint symptoms who experience a limitation in activity due to arthritis.
- Reduce activity limitations due to chronic back conditions.

Heart Diseases and Stroke
- Reduce coronary heart disease deaths.
- Reduce stroke deaths.
- Reduce the proportion of adults with high blood pressure.

Nutrition and Overweight
- Increase the proportion of adults who are at a healthy weight.
- Reduce the proportion of children and adolescents who are overweight or obese.
- Increase the proportion of persons aged two years and older who consume at least two daily servings of fruit.

Physical Fitness and Activity
- Increase the proportion of adults who engage regularly, preferably daily, in moderate physical activity for at least 30 minutes.
- Increase the proportion of the nation's public and private schools that require daily physical education for all students.

Substance Abuse
- Reduce deaths and injuries caused by alcohol- and drug-related motor vehicle crashes.
- Reduce cirrhosis deaths.
- Reduce the proportion of persons engaging in binge drinking of alcoholic beverages.
- Reduce past month use of illicit substances.

Tobacco Use
- Reduce tobacco use by adults and adolescents.
- Increase smoking cessation during pregnancy.
- Reduce the proportion of children who are regularly exposed to tobacco smoke at home.
- Reduce the illegal sale rate to minors through enforcement of laws prohibiting the sale of tobacco products to minors.

Environmental Health
- Reduce the proportion of persons exposed to air that does not meet the U.S. Environmental Protection Agency's health-based standards for harmful air pollutants.
- Eliminate elevated blood lead levels in children.
- Reduce waterborne disease outbreaks arising from water intended for drinking among persons served by community water systems.

Source: Adapted from U.S. Department of Health and Human Services, *Healthy People 2010: Understanding and Improving Health* (Washington, DC: U.S. Government Printing Office, January 2000).

combination of the two, with genetics and lifestyle both playing important roles in determining a child's weight. Our society has become sedentary. Television, computers, and video games contribute to inactive lifestyles for children and adults. Forty-three percent of adolescents watch more than two hours of television each day.

According to the Surgeon General, approximately 300,000 deaths in the United States each year may be

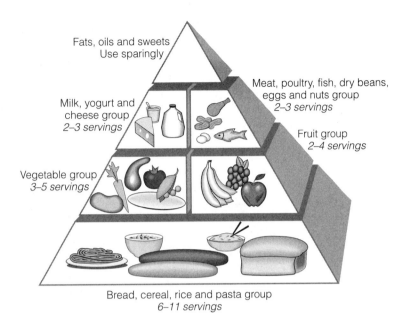

Fats, oils and sweets
Use sparingly

Meat, poultry, fish, dry beans,
eggs and nuts group
2–3 servings

Milk, yogurt and
cheese group
2–3 servings

Fruit group
2–4 servings

Vegetable group
3–5 servings

Bread, cereal, rice and pasta group
6–11 servings

Figure 10.4 Food Guide Pyramid: A guide to daily food choices.

attributable to obesity. Overweight and obesity are associated with heart disease, certain types of cancer, type 2 diabetes, stroke, arthritis, breathing problems, and psychological disorders such as depression.

Increase in Obesity

- 11–25 percent of U.S. children and teens are obese.

- One child in three is now either obese or at risk for becoming so.

- According to the Centers for Disease Control and Prevention (CDC), the number of obese Americans increased by 60 percent between 1991 and 1999.

- From 1991 to 1998, more states report high obesity rates.

- More than 60 percent of U.S. residents are overweight; nearly 50 percent are obese.

- Physical inactivity contributes to childhood obesity.

Health Risks

- Obesity in children increases their risk of cardiovascular disease.

- Obesity in children increases risk of other diseases, including diabetes.

- The increase in diabetes over the past decade is alarming— it has increased 70 percent in people in their thirties.

- The overall increase in diabetes nationwide is 33 percent (but that is probably an underestimate).

Diabetes and Obesity

- Type 2 diabetes, previously considered an adult disease, has increased dramatically in children and adolescents. Overweight and obesity are closely linked to type 2 diabetes.

- More than 80 percent of people with diabetes are overweight or obese.

Adolescents and Adults

- Overweight adolescents have a 70 percent chance of becoming overweight or obese adults. This increases to 80 percent if at least one parent is overweight or obese.

Physical activity is the key to reducing obesity and diabetes in children. Therefore, each student in grades K–12 should take physical education instruction each school day. State boards of education should adopt necessary rules and methods to implement this requirement.

CHANGING DEMOGRAPHICS OF THE UNITED STATES

The demographics of American society is rapidly changing, as is evident in the aging population, the disabled population, cultural and ethnic diversity, and family structure.

Aging Population

The U.S. population is shifting from a younger generation to an older generation, and this trend is expected to continue. The U.S. life expectancy averages seventy-seven years (seventy-three for men and eighty for women). In 2000,

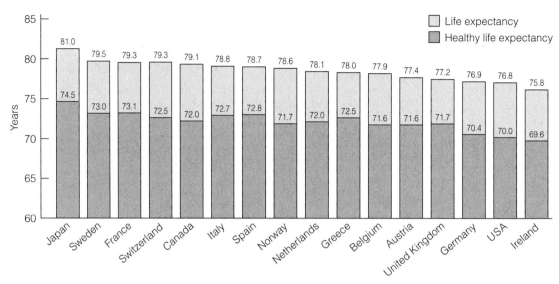

Figure 10.5 Life expectancy estimates for selected countries.

the World Health Organization (WHO), for the first time, calculated **healthy life expectancy (HLE)** estimates for 191 nations. The United States ranked twenty-fourth in this report, with an HLE of 70 years. Japan was first with an HLE of 74.5 years (see Figure 10.5).

The average age of Americans this decade is dramatically higher than the average age in the last decade. In 1900, approximately 3.1 percent of the population was sixty-five and older. In 1993, 32.3 percent of the population was within this age group, and in 2000, it was 35.3 percent. It is estimated that in 2010, it will be 40.1 percent; in 2020, 53.3 percent; and in 2030, 70.2 percent. In addition, these older people are expected to be very healthy. In terms of actual numbers, rather than percentages, in 1999 there were 34.5 million older adults age sixty-five and over in the United States. This represents about one in every eight Americans. In 1996, the number of people eighty-five years and older was 3.8 million, and it will be more than 7 million in 2025.

Advances in technology and medicine will help Americans live a longer and more productive life. Cures for AIDS, cancer (colon, rectum, breast, lung), diabetes, heart disease, and other diseases will lengthen life. With more free time

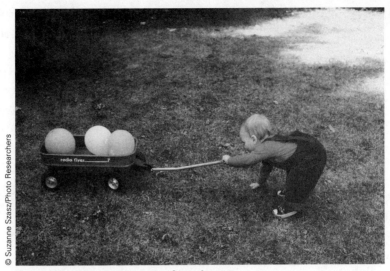

You are never too young to enjoy physical activity.

available and a longer life, older adults will seek lifetime recreational activities that will prevent degeneration and disease and will enhance their health and well-being. In the future, quality health and physical activity programs will increase for the growing population of older adults.

Americans with Disabilities

The current trend in physical education is to place students in the least restrictive environment (LRE), which requires that all students be placed in a setting that will result in the best opportunity for success and educational progress. Debates will continue in the twenty-first century about the pros and cons of **inclusion,** the philosophy of merging special and general education and placing all children with disabilities in a general education setting. Some published reports indicate inclusion in physical education can be successful, but stories from practicing physical educators also indicate inclusion does not always work. To some extent, the problems occur because inclusion is not being carried out properly. Students with disabilities are "dumped" into general physical education without providing any staff training or support to the physical educator or adapted physical educator; other problems are large class size, lack of individualized information, class management problems, and the reluctance of many physical education teachers to work with these children.

The current trend is that more communities are abandoning the philosophy of inclusion and are going back to more special classrooms and special schools for children with disabilities. However, recent reauthorization of the Individuals with Disabilities Act (IDEA) and recent court interpretations of least restrictive environment suggest that the legal system favors inclusion.

Cultural and Ethnic Diversity

The American population is becoming more diverse as the number of African American, Hispanic, Asian, and Native American citizens has increased. **Diversity** is a fact of American life; education can help promote understanding and acceptance of diverse viewpoints and **cultures.** Cultural dialogue helps promote respect for individuality, mutual acceptance, and recognition of human rights.

Physical education programs can help break down barriers of cultural and language differences. Everyone likes to play and to have fun. The study of cultural, linguistic, and **ethnic** differences will begin early in a student's education in order to celebrate **multiculturalism** and preserve wisdom and uniqueness.

The Hispanic population in the United States was 24 million in 1996. By the year 2010, Hispanics will be the largest ethnic minority, surpassing African Americans. It is anticipated that, by the year 2050, the U.S. population will be evenly divided in thirds among Hispanics, non-Hispanic whites, and other ethnic groups. By 2020, Hispanics combined with other ethnic minorities in the school-aged population will represent approximately 45 percent of the school-aged population, with 55 percent represented by non-Hispanic whites.

Ethnic minorities are projected to represent 25 percent of the population sixty-five and older in 2030, compared to 13 percent in 1996. Between 1990 and 2030, the older non-Hispanic white population is projected to increase tremendously. The number of older Hispanics will increase by more than the number of non-Hispanic blacks. The number of Native Americans, Asians, and Pacific Islanders will also increase. The numbers of cultural and ethnic minority graduates with specializations in fitness, health education, and other related physical education disciplines are projected to increase. Due to the increase in cultural and ethnic minority groups, more minority teachers will be hired to serve as role models and mentors for an increasing number of ethnically diverse students. College students will be more career-oriented, older, and diverse in background.

Family Structures

The number of teenage mothers, single-parent families, dual-career families, and families headed by guardians such as grandparents and other relatives has led to "latchkey" and "couch potato" children—children who come home at the end of the school day, often to be alone for hours, and turn on the television or computer. Thanks in part to these devices, children are becoming less active and more overweight than previous generations were. Changes in the family have meant a growing concern for the safety of children, as well as concern for their sedentary lifestyle, for children are being exposed to drug and alcohol abuse, risky sexual behaviors, child abuse, and violence.

Day care and after-school programs will expand in the future. The physical educator must be prepared to conduct quality physical activity programs and provide recreational opportunities within as well as outside the school setting.

PHYSICAL EDUCATION IN THE TWENTY-FIRST CENTURY

School and Higher Education Programs

In the twenty-first century the physical education curriculum in elementary and secondary schools will emphasize technology, physical fitness, skill development and maintenance, as well as **health-enhancing skills, interactive behavior** (social and emotional health), and **motor skills.** In order to ensure quality of physical education programs and to save money due to cutbacks in school funding, local school systems may employ outside agencies to deliver programs that emphasize health issues (obesity, blood pressure, cardiovascular disease, diabetes). Accountability will lead physical educators to establish national standards for student achievement through performance assessment. In addition, accountability will ensure that physical educators will upgrade their instructional skills and content knowledge by attending in-service workshops and conferences. An increased number of cultural and ethnic minority teachers will be employed to serve as role models for the increasingly diverse population. Knowledge of subject and performance skills will determine merit pay and other rewards to recognize excellence. Those who wish to become physical educators will be required to take competency exams. To enhance programs that are appropriate to the developmental needs of students, teachers will incorporate technology and computer skills.

College physical education professors will be required to keep abreast of the knowledge, skills, and technology required to be specialists in physical education. College instructors will specialize in the applied sciences and **brain-based instruction.** Research productivity will continue to be a standard for promotion and tenure. Cultural and ethnic minorities will be recruited to the faculty to serve as mentors for a diverse student body.

The number of physical education graduates will increase, especially those with specializations in fitness, health education promotion, exercise physiology, sports management, and athletic training. Five-year teacher education programs will become the standard, while certifications and advanced education will be required of sport and exercise practitioners. Elective physical education activity programs focusing on weight training, outdoor leisure pursuits, aerobic activities and lifetime sport will become more popular than the standard physical education classes consisting of sport skills.

Physical Activity and Fitness Programs

Physical activity and fitness programs will continue to increase at a rapid rate in the twenty-first century. More con-

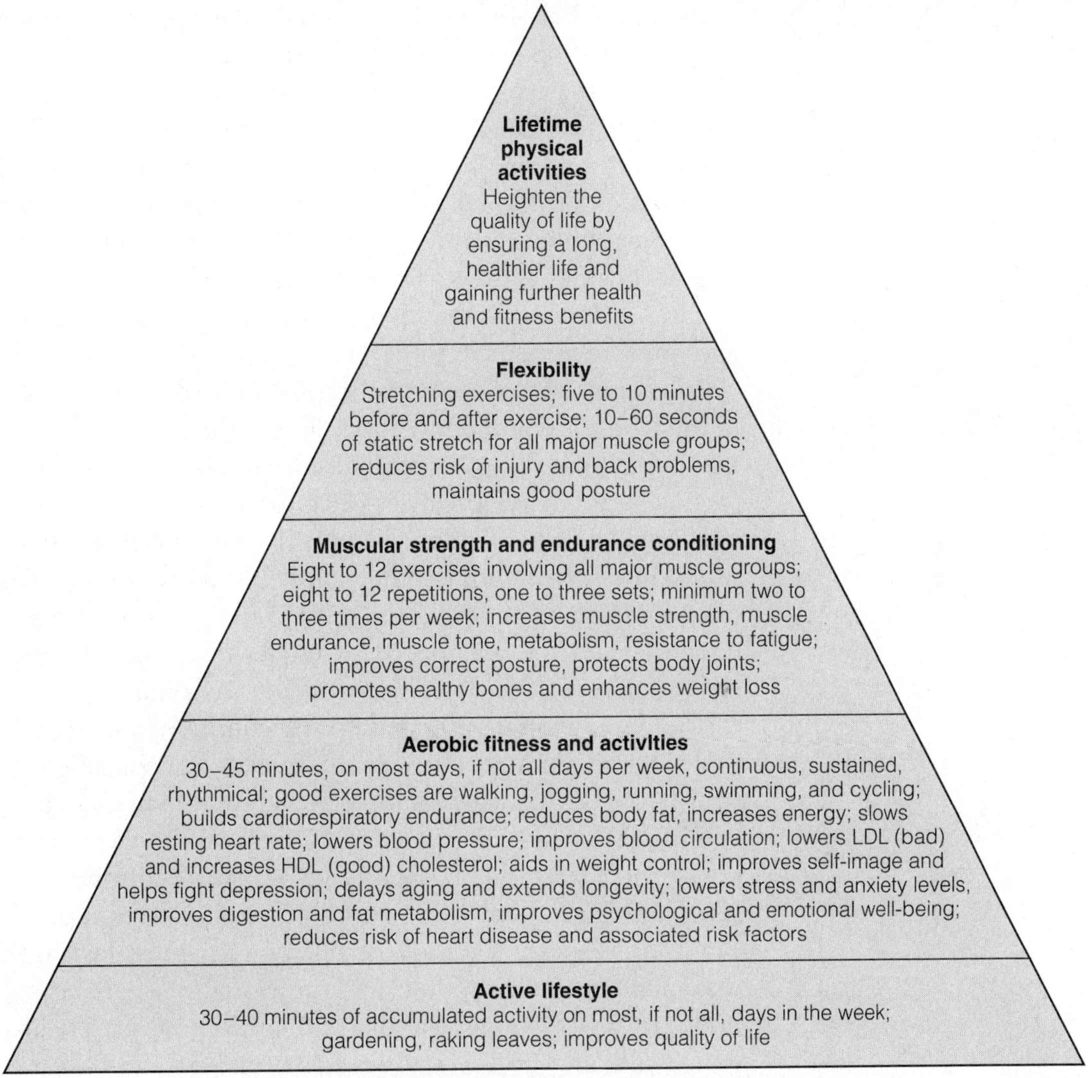

Lifetime physical activities
Heighten the quality of life by ensuring a long, healthier life and gaining further health and fitness benefits

Flexibility
Stretching exercises; five to 10 minutes before and after exercise; 10–60 seconds of static stretch for all major muscle groups; reduces risk of injury and back problems, maintains good posture

Muscular strength and endurance conditioning
Eight to 12 exercises involving all major muscle groups; eight to 12 repetitions, one to three sets; minimum two to three times per week; increases muscle strength, muscle endurance, muscle tone, metabolism, resistance to fatigue; improves correct posture, protects body joints; promotes healthy bones and enhances weight loss

Aerobic fitness and activities
30–45 minutes, on most days, if not all days per week, continuous, sustained, rhythmical; good exercises are walking, jogging, running, swimming, and cycling; builds cardiorespiratory endurance; reduces body fat, increases energy; slows resting heart rate; lowers blood pressure; improves blood circulation; lowers LDL (bad) and increases HDL (good) cholesterol; aids in weight control; improves self-image and helps fight depression; delays aging and extends longevity; lowers stress and anxiety levels, improves digestion and fat metabolism, improves psychological and emotional well-being; reduces risk of heart disease and associated risk factors

Active lifestyle
30–40 minutes of accumulated activity on most, if not all, days in the week; gardening, raking leaves; improves quality of life

Note: Please consult a physician before beginning any physical activity program

Figure 10.6 Physical Activity Pyramid.

tent and skills knowledge will be required of those earning bachelor's and master's degrees, and advanced certifications will be required of fitness instructors and managers in fitness centers. Physical educators will become proactive in directing community fitness programs. Corporations will continue to expand on fitness and wellness programs for employees. Corporate investment in these programs is evidence that corporations believe that fitness and wellness programs result in increased employee productivity, decreased absenteeism, lower insurance costs, and better employee health. Fitness instructors and managers will continue to assist youth and adults in developing healthy lifestyles by changing their participation levels. Older-adult fitness programs and outdoor recreational activities will rapidly increase and attract new participants. After-school physical activity programs for children, adolescents, and parents will increase and encourage youth to remain active.

Consumers will continue to become more discriminating in their fitness equipment, apparel, selection of activities, and nutritional choices to reduce calories, fat, and cholesterol. Technological advances will allow participants to enhance skill and performances and will dramatically change fitness and sports equipment, facilities, and programs. Sales of home exercise equipment, apparel, and sporting goods equipment will be phenomenally higher than in the twentieth century. With the latest medical advice from experts in the field, individual participation will continue to increase and become the American way of life. Physical education professionals will assume a more proactive role in the leadership of the physical activity and fitness programs among youth and adults not only in the school but also in the nonschool setting. There will be more physical education programs to meet the needs of the very young, individuals with disabilities, and older adults and individuals who are economically disadvantaged and lack financial resources to afford health and fitness facilities.

Technology

Today's physical education teachers are being prepared to effectively integrate technology into their classes and provide technologically supported learning opportunities for their students.

The physical educator can use word-processing software, spreadsheets and database software, desktop publishing software, graphics software, and multimedia software such as PowerPoint and Hyperstudio. On the Internet, newsgroups, email, and email discussion groups allow physical educators to communicate and collaborate with colleagues worldwide. **Newsgroups** are discussion forums on specific topics. Participants can read all messages and replies between the participants; newsgroups are public and available to anyone with an Internet connection. You can think of a newsgroup as an electronic bulletin board. **Email** is a quick method of sending and receiving messages using computer mail programs and an Internet connection; today email can increasingly be accessed via a Web browser as well as a traditional mail program. **Electronic mailing lists** (or email discussion groups) are discussion groups that provide a forum for people with common interests to pose questions, engage in discussions, and share their views. Messages are distributed through email to a list of subscribers who respond to the discussion topic. Many mailing lists are open to anyone; others require approval of a moderator, and some limit membership to retain a "small-group" feeling.

Internet telephones and videoconferencing will enhance communications with colleagues worldwide. **Distance learning** will continue to use the Web and desktop videoconferencing. Continuing education programs offered through distance learning will allow one-to-one teaching and learning; courses and degrees will be completed via the Internet, television, and other technological methods. For example, a teacher in California can participate in a workshop on physical education hosted by the American Alliance for Health, Physical Education, Recreation and Dance (AAHPERD) in Reston, Virginia, and receive college credit. Hardware, such as heart rate monitors, fat analyzers, pulse counters, pedometers, handheld personal computers, and digital recorders and cameras will continuously be improved for use in physical education.

Virtual reality offers opportunities for training and lessons in physical education. Virtual reality uses computers and sensory mechanisms to create simulated, interactive three-dimensional environments. A game or simulation, using sensor gloves and head-mounted displays, can be a part of virtual reality in the typical physical education classroom. Virtual reality places the participant's body inside the three-dimensional environment. The participant experiences a real-life situation by reacting to changing scenarios. Today, virtual reality is used for sports such as bobsledding, baseball, football, and golf to improve the athlete's performance. As technology becomes more advanced, virtual reality will be more cost-effective and will be used more frequently in physical education and physical activity programs.

The traditional educational practices are no longer sufficient for teaching students. Multimedia and the World Wide Web have made interactive learning and global communication essential to the educational process. Technological innovations will continue to improve, and teachers must challenge their students to become active and lifelong learners who are prepared to meet the demands of a rapidly changing society.

Physical Education and Service Learning

In order for physical education to remain relevant, physical educators must serve populations in school and nonschool settings. Physical educators must be more responsive to health advances in order to help students get and remain fit and healthy. Prevention of disease through achievement of fitness is the key to the future of physical education. By keeping fit, healthy students will not develop or will reduce the risk of hypokinetic (lack of activity) diseases or conditions such as cardiovascular disease, obesity, type 2 diabetes, hypertension, and high cholesterol.

To promote cost-effectiveness, school physical education programs will continue to share facilities, equipment, personnel, and activities with community programs. This conjunction will help provide a progression of activities throughout life for all ages. More communities will provide and promote the use of safe, well-maintained, and close-to-home sidewalks, bike paths, trails, and recreation facilities.

Technology will help physical educators provide individual instruction to meet the program needs of a diverse and aging population. Telecommunication networking will make possible collaborative research endeavors with colleagues worldwide. Distance and cooperative learning, video, and cable television will offer students step-by step approaches to gaining knowledge and skills in physical activities so that they can maintain and improve their physical fitness and activity levels. The use of digital cameras, videotape, spreadsheets, databases, and hypermedia presentations will allow feedback on individual performances and help individuals improve their motor skills and maintain progress toward the attainment of their goals.

THE FUTURE OF PHYSICAL EDUCATION

The challenges for the physical education professional are numerous. Those preparing to become physical educators should maintain an excellent grade-point average and continue the study of present trends and their relationship to careers in physical education. The public's search for healthy lifestyle through physical activity will be best served if physical education and physical activity professionals are leading, rather than reacting to, the latest trends.

We hope that as you have read and studied this textbook, we have helped you to develop your personal and professional goals and to understand the profession of physical education. As a future physical education professional, you will help ensure that physical education and physical activity programs are accepted and advanced.

Physical education professionals can determine the future of physical education. In order to meet demands of the future, physical educators must

- Be dedicated and committed professionals
- Take charge of their professional destiny
- Obtain proper credentials and claim their domain by seeking leadership positions
- Integrate technology in their daily lives
- Provide physical activities for healthier living to all populations, regardless of age, disabling conditions, and socioeconomic conditions
- Realize that individuals will live longer and must be fit and active in these years
- Accept only excellence in all their professional endeavors

- Encourage and provide recommendations for women and ethnic and cultural minorities in leadership positions

- Serve as positive role models for a fit and healthy lifestyle so others will follow

- Make a commitment to have high-quality developmental programs for the young as well as the older adults.

Physical education has a very promising future and has tremendous potential to enhance the health and quality of life for all Americans. It is left up to each of us as physical education professionals to make a personal commitment to excellence. We have a tremendous past to inspire us, the present to sustain us, and the future to challenge us. We, the authors of this text, challenge you, as young professionals of physical education, to lead us into a promising and healthy future in the profession in which we serve.

On the Web

http://www.eatright.org
This American Dietetic Association site includes a vast amount of information on nutrition.

http://www.nal.usda.gov/fnic/dga/index.html
Dietary Guidelines from the Food and Nutrition Information Center. This site features Dietary Guidelines for Americans, 2000, and links to historical dietary guidelines and dietary guidelines from twenty countries.

http://www.healthypeople.gov/
Healthy People 2010. Healthy People is a national health promotion and disease prevention initiative that lists a series of goals for improving the health of all Americans by 2010.

http://www.nal.usda.gov:8001/py/pmap.htm
The Interactive Food Guide Pyramid. This site allows you to select different components of the Food Guide Pyramid to learn how to incorporate the proper nutrients into your daily diet.

http://www.pbs.org/als/teach_students
This site and those in the following list provide information on teaching students with special needs.

http://www.newhorizons.org

http://www.palaestra.com/Inclusion.html

http://www.specialolympics.org/

http://www.paralympic.org

http://www.disabledsports.org/

http://www.creativeimaginations.net

Key Terms

brain-based instruction Teaching and curriculum based on the way the brain works. The physical education classroom is highly brain-compatible: It offers the stimulation, repetition, and novelty that enhance learning (page 244).

culture The sum total of ways of living that have evolved for a group of human beings and have been transmitted from one group to another. A collection of individual life experiences; includes ethnicity, religion, gender, interests, activities, abilities, social class, professions, customs, and lifestyles (page 242).

distance learning Education delivered via video or computer to students who are not in the same location as the teacher—in fact, who are anywhere in the world (page 247).

diversity The state of having varied, and unlike, qualities or elements (page 242).

electronic mailing lists Private discussion groups that provide a forum, via the Internet, for people with common interests to pose questions, engage in discussions, and share their views. Messages are exchanged via email; participation requires "subscription," which may be limited and require approval by a "moderator." Some electronic mailing lists are open to anyone (page 247).

email A quick method of sending and receiving messages via computer and an Internet connection (page 247).

ethnic Pertaining to groups of people categorized according to shared national, religious, linguistic, or cultural origin or background (page 242).

Food Guide Pyramid An aid to following fitness guidelines; it groups foods into six categories, indicating serving sizes for each (page 235).

health-enhancing skills Regular physical activity that results in substantial improvements in health and well-being. Health-related fitness components include cardiovascular efficiency, muscular strength, muscular endurance, flexibility, and body composition (page 243).

healthy life expectancy (HLE) Refers to the number of years a person is expected to live in good health. This number is obtained by subtracting ill-health years from the overall life expectancy (page 240).

inclusion The philosophy of merging special and general education and placing all children with disabilities in a general education setting (page 241).

interactive behavior Refers to safe practices, adherence to rules and procedures, etiquette, cooperation, teamwork, ethical behavior in sports, and positive social interaction when participating in physical activity. Also includes the intrinsic value and benefits of participation in physical activity (page 243).

motor skills Refers to the basic fundamental movement patterns that are necessary to perform a variety of physical activities. Consists of locomotor, nonlocomotor, and manipulative skills (page 243).

multiculturalism Respect for and integration of various cultures (page 242).

newsgroups Public discussion forums on specific topics, with all messages posted (as on a bulletin board) for users to view. Anyone with Internet access can read all messages and replies between the participants (page 247).

Physical Activity Pyramid Grouping of physical activity guidelines into five categories, with recommendations for each category (page 245).

virtual reality Using the computers and sensory mechanisms to create simulated, interactive three-dimensional environments (page 247).

Multiple Choice Questions

1. Private discussion groups conducted via email that provide a forum for people with common interests to pose questions, engage in discussions, and share their views.
   a. electronic mailing lists
   b. Web forums
   c. voice mail
   d. newsgroups

2. A method of sending and receiving messages via a computer
   a. virtual reality
   b. email
   c. distance learning
   d. voice mail

3. Using the computers and sensory mechanisms to create simulated, interactive three-dimensional environments
   a. distance learning
   b. computer assisted instruction (CSI)
   c. virtual reality
   d. computer based instruction (CBI)

4. The sum total of ways of living that have evolved for a group of human beings and have been transmitted from one group to another refers to

   a. ethnicity
   b. culture
   c. diversity
   d. multiculturalism

5. Public discussion forums on specific topics; all messages and replies are available to anyone with Internet access.

   a. electronic mailing lists
   b. virtual reality
   c. computer assisted instruction (CAI)
   d. newsgroups

6. The curriculum goal which refers to regular physical activity that results in substantial improvements in health and well-being is known as

   a. motor skill development
   b. interactive behavior
   c. health-enhancing physical activity
   d. healthy life expectancy (HLE)

7. The curriculum goal that refers to safe practices, adherence to rules and procedures, etiquette, cooperation, teamwork, ethical behavior in sports, and positive social interaction when participating in physical activity is

   a. motor skill development
   b. interactive behavior
   c. health-enhancing physical activity
   d. healthy life expectancy (HLE)

8. The curriculum goal which refers to the basic fundamental movement patterns that are necessary to perform a variety of physical activities. Consists of locomotor, nonlocomotor, and manipulative skills.

   a. motor skill development
   b. interactive behavior
   c. health-enhancing behavior
   d. healthy life expectancy (HLE)

9. What is the key to promoting, understanding, and accepting diversity?

   a. people
   b. minorities
   c. education
   d. cultural diversity

10. Education delivered to students who are in a different location from the instructor is known as

   a. inquiry based learning
   b. critical thinking
   c. cooperative learning
   d. distance learning

Critical Thinking Questions

1. Identify at least three trends that will influence society and you as a physical education professional during the twenty-first century. How would you like to shape these trends? What direction would you like to see them take?

2. Explain how technology will affect physical education and physical activity programs in the future.

3. Describe changes that are projected for school physical education programs in the twenty-first century.

4. Discuss the need for more physical activity and recreational programs for older adults. Why are these programs essential in the twenty-first century?

5. Discuss the changes that you predict for physical education in 2010? 2030? 2050? What is the greatest challenge that you expect to confront during your teaching career in this decade? How will you meet this challenge?

References

Auxter, D., Pyfer, J., and Huettig C. *Principles and Methods of Adapted Physical Education and Recreation with Gross Motor Activities* 9th ed. St. Louis, Mo.: Mosby: 2001.

Block, M. E. "Did We Jump on the Wrong Bandwagon? Making General Physical Education Placement Work." *Palaestra*, 13, no. 3 (1999): 34–42.

Block, M. E. "Did We Jump on the Wrong Bandwagon? Problems with Inclusion in Physical Education." *Palaestra*, 13, no. 2 (1999): 30–36, 55–56.

Block, M. E. *A Teacher's Guide to Including Students with Disabilities in Regular Physical Education*, 2nd. ed. Baltimore, Md.: Paul H. Brookes, 2000.

Blubaugh, Donelle. "Bringing Cable into the Classroom." *Educational Leadership*, 56, no. 5: (1999): 61–65.

Corbin, David E., and Josie Metal-Corbin. *Reach for It: A Handbook for Health, Exercise & Dance Activities for Older Adults*, 3rd. ed. Peosta, Iowa: Eddie Bowers, 1997.

Floyd, Patricia A., and Allen, Beverly J. *Professional Preparation of Pre-Service Teachers*. Boston, Mass.: Pearson Education, 2003.

Floyd, Patricia, Mimms, Sandra, and Yelding, Caroline. *Personal Health: Perspectives and Lifestyles*, 3rd. ed. Belmont, Calif.: Wadsworth, 2003.

Haggerty, T. R. "Influence of Information Technologies on Kinesiology and Physical Education," *Quest* 49 (1997): 254–269.

Hoeger, Werner W. K., Turner, Lori W., Hafen, Brent Q. *Wellness: Guideline for a Healthy Lifestyle*, 3rd. ed. Belmont, Calif.: Wadsworth, 2002.

Lumpkin, Angela *Physical Education and Sport: A Contemporary Introduction*, 5th ed. Boston, Mass.: WCB McGraw-Hill, 2002.

Public Health Service, U.S Department of Health and Human Services. *Healthy People 2010: National Health Promotion and Disease Prevention Objectives*. Washington, D.C., U.S. Government Printing Office.

Rutledge, Earl. *Trends in Educational Technology. Eric Digest*. 1995. http://www.coe.iup.edu/med_distance/633/technolo.htm (August 27, 2000).

U.S. Administration on Aging and American Association of Retired Persons. *A Profile of Older Americans. 1997*. Washington D.C.: U.S. Government Printing Office, 1997.

U.S. Department of Health and Human Services, Centers for Disease Control and Prevention, *Deaths: Final Data for 1998*, 48, no. 11 (July 23, 2000).

U.S. Department of Health and Human Services. *Physical Activity and Health: A Report of the Surgeon General*. Atlanta, Ga.: Centers for Disease Control and Prevention, National Center for Chronic Disease Prevention and Health Promotion, 1996.

U.S. Department of Health, Education, and Welfare*: Healthy People: The Surgeon General's Report on Health Promotion and Disease Prevention*. Washington, D.C.: U.S. Government Printing Office, 1979.

World Health Organization, Ch-1211 Geneva 27, Switzerland.

Wuest, Deborah A., and Bucher, Charles A. *Foundations of Physical Education and Sport*, 13th ed. Boston, Mass.: WCB/McGraw-Hill, 1999.

APPENDIX A

Professional Organizations Relating to Physical Education and Sport

Note that many organizations have email directories on their Web sites. Information may change, and updates can be found with an Internet search engine.

DANCE ORGANIZATIONS

National Dance Association
1900 Association Drive
Reston, VA 20191
Phone: 800-213-7193, Ext. 464
Web site: http://www.aahperd.org/nda

PE Central
P.O. Box 10262
Blacksburg, VA 24062
Phone: 540-953-1043
Fax: 800-783-8124
Email: pec@pecentral.org
Note: PE Central Web site, http://www.pecentral.org, has links to numerous dance sites.

United States Amateur Ballroom Dancers Association
P.O. Box 128
New Freedom, PA 17349
Phone: 800-447-9047
Fax: 717-235-4183
Email: Usabdacent@aol.com
Web site: http://www.usabda.org

Additional Web Sites for Dance:
Line Dance: http://hometown.aol.com/pbrown4715/dance1.htm
Step Aerobics: http://www.turnstep.com
Dance Directory: http://www.SapphireSwan.com/dance
Tap Dance: http://www.tapdance.org/tap
Ballroom: http://www.ballroomdancers.com

EDUCATION ORGANIZATIONS

Cooper Institute for Aerobics Research
12330 Preston Road
Dallas, TX 75230
Phone: 972-341-3200
              800-635-7050
Fax: 972-341-3227
Web site: http://www.cooperinst.org

International Diabetic Athletes Association
P.O. Box 1935
Litchfield Park, AZ 85340
Phone: 623-535-4593
             800-898-4322
Fax: 623-535-4741
Email: desa@diabetes-exercise.org
Web site: http://www.diabetes-exercise.org

National Association for Sports and Physical Education
1900 Association Drive
Reston, VA 20191
Phone: 800-213-7193, Ext. 410
Email: naspe@aahperd.org
Web site: http://www.aahperd.org/naspe

National Coalition for Promoting Physical Activity
1010 Massachusetts Ave., Suite 350
Washington, D.C. 20001
Phone: 202-454-7521
Fax: 202-454-7598
Email: info@ncppa.org
Web site: http://www.ncppa.org

National Safety Council
1121 Spring Lake Drive
Itasca, IL 60143-3201
Phone: 630-285-1121
Fax: 630-285-1315
Email: info@nsc.org
Web site: http://www.nsc.org

The Society for Public Health Education, Inc.
750 First St. NE, Suite 910
Washington, DC 20002-4242
Phone   202-408-9804
Email: info@sophe.org
Web site: http://www.sophe.org

Wilderness Medical Society
3595 E. Fountain Blvd., Suite 1
Colorado Springs, CO 80910
Phone: 719-572-9255
Fax: 719-572-1514
Email: wms@wms.org
Web site: http://www.wms.org

HEALTH ORGANIZATIONS

Aerobics and Fitness Association of America
15250 Ventura Boulevard, Suite 200
Sherman Oaks, CA 91403
Phone: 877-968-7263
Fax: 818-788-6301
Email: ContactAFAA@afaa.com
Web site: http://www.afaa.com

American Academy of Family Physicians
P.O. Box 11210
Shawnee Mission, KS 66207-1210
Phone: 800-274-2237
Web site: http://www.aafp.org

American Academy of Orthopedic Surgeons
6300 North River Road
Rosemont, IL 60018-4263
Phone: 847-823-7186
              800-346-AAOS
Fax: 847-823-8125
Web site: http://www.aaos.org

American Academy of Physical Medicine & Rehabilitation
One IBM Plaza, Suite 2500
Chicago, IL 60611-3604
Phone: 312-464-9700
Fax: 312-464-0227
Email: info@aapmr.org
Web site: http://www.aapmr.org

American Alliance for Health, Physical Education, Recreation and Dance/American Association for Active Lifestyles and Fitness (AAHPERD/AAALF)
1900 Association Drive
Reston, VA 20191
Phone: 800-213-7193
Email: Info@aahperd.org
Web site: http://www.aahperd.org/

American Association for Health Education
1900 Association Drive
Reston, VA 20191
Phone: 800-213-7193, Ext. 437
Email: aahe@aahperd.org
Web site: http://www.aahperd.org/aahe

**American Association of Cardiovascular
and Pulmonary Rehabilitation**
401 North Michigan Avenue
Suite 2200
Chicago, IL 60611
Phone: 312-321-5146
Fax: 312-527-6635
Email: aacvpr@sba.com
Web site: http://www.aacvpr.org

American Association of Occupational Health
2920 Brandywine Road, Suite 100
Atlanta, GA 30341
Phone: 770-455-7757
Fax: 770-455-7271
Email: aaohn@aaohn.org
Web site: http://www.aaohn.org

American College of Cardiology
9111 Old Georgetown Road
Bethesda, MD 20814
Phone: 301-897-5400
             800-253-4636, ext. 694
Fax: 301-897-9745
Email: resource@acc.org
Web site: http://www.acc.org

American College of Sports Medicine (ACSM)
P.O. Box 1440
Indianapolis, IN 46206-1440
Phone: 317-637-9200
Fax: 317-634-7817
Web site: http://www.acsm.org

American Council on Exercise (ACE)
4851 Paramount Drive
San Diego, California 92123
Phone: 858-279-8227
             800-825-3636
Fax: 858-279-8064
Web site: http://www.acefitness.org

American Council on Science and Health
1995 Broadway, Second Floor
New York, NY 10023-5860
Phone: 212-362-7044
Fax: 212-362-4919
Email: acsh@acsh.org
Web site: http://www.acsh.org

American Heart Association
7272 Greenville Ave.
Dallas, TX 75231-4592
Phone: 800-242-8721
Web site: http://www.americanheart.org

American Kinesiotherapy Association
One IBM Plaza, Suite 2500
Chicago, IL 60611
Phone: 800-296-2582
Fax: 312-464-2007
Web site: http://www.akta.org

American Medical Society for Sports Medicine (AMSSM)
11639 Earnshaw
Overland Park, KS 66210
Phone: 913-327-1415
Fax: 913-327-1491
Email: office@amssm.org
Web site: http://www.amssm.org

American Occupational Therapy Association
4720 Montgomery Lane
PO Box 31220
Bethesda, MD 20824-1220
Phone 301-652-2682
Fax 301-652-7711
Web site: http://www.aota.org

American Orthopaedic Society for Sports Medicine
6300 North River Road, Suite 500
Rosemont, IL 60018
Phone: 847-292-4900
Fax: 847-292-4905
Web site: http://www.sportsmed.org

American Physical Therapy Association
11111 North Fairfax Street
Alexandria, VA 22314
Phone: 703-684-2782
        800-999-2782
Fax: 703-684-7343
Web site: http://www.apta.org

American Public Health Association
800 I Street NW
Washington, DC 20001
Phone: 202-777-2742
Fax: 202-777-2534
Email: comments@apha.org
Web site: http://www.apha.org

American Society of Biomechanics
2450 Lozana Road
Delmar, CA 92014
Phone: 401-444-4231

Aquatic Exercise Association
3439 Technology Drive, Suite 6
Nakomis, FL 34275-3627
Phone: 941-486-8600
            888-AEA-WAVE
Fax: 941-486-8820
Email: info@aeawave.com
Web site: http://www.aeawave.com

Arthritis Foundation
P.O. Box 7669
Atlanta, GA 30357-0669
Phone: 800-283-7800
Web site: http://www.arthritis.org

Association for Community Health Improvement
2119 Mapleton Avenue
Boulder, CO 80304
Phone: 303-444-3366
Email: healthy@aha.org
Web: site: http://www.healthycommunities.org

Association of Schools of Public Health (ASPH)
1101 15th Street NW Suite 910
Washington DC 20005
Phone: 202-296-1099
Fax: 202-296-1252
Email: info@asph.org
Web site http://www.asph.org

Association of State Territorial Health Officials
1275 K Street NW Suite. 800
Washington. DC 20005-4006
Phone: 202-371-9090
Fax: 202-371-9797
Web site: http://www.astho.org

Citizens for Public Action on
High Blood Pressure and Cholesterol
P.O. Box 30374
Bethesda, MD 20824
Phone: 301-770-1711
Fax: 301-770-1713

Healthy People 2010
Office of Disease Prevention and Health Promotion
Humphrey Bldg., Room 738-G
200 Independence Ave. SW
Washington, DC 20201
Fax: 202-205-9478
Email: hp2010@osophs.dhhs.gov
Web site: http://www.healthypeople.gov

IDEA, The International Association of Fitness Professionals
6190 Cornerstone Court E., Suite 204
San Diego, CA 92121
Phone: 800-999-4332
Fax: 610-535-8234
Email: nonmemberquestions@ideafit.com
Web site: http://www.ideafit.com

The Leukemia and Lymphoma Society
1311 Mamaroneck Ave.
White Plains, NY 10605
Phone: 914-949-5213
          800-955-4572
Fax   914-949-6691
Web site: http://www.leukemia.org

**National Arthritis & Musculoskeletal and
Skin Disease Information Clearing House**
National Institutes of Health
1 AMS Circle
Bethesda, Maryland 20892-3675
Phone: 301-495-4484
          877-22-NIAMS
Fax: 301-718-6366
Email: niamsinfo@mail.nih.gov
Web site: http://www.nih.gov/niams

**The National Association for Health & Fitness—
The Network of State and Governor's Councils**
401 W. Michigan Street
Indianapolis, IN 46202-3233
Phone: 317-955-0957
Fax: 317-634-7817
Email: info@physicalfitness.org
Web site: http://www.physicalfitness.org

National Center for Chronic Disease Prevention and Health Promotion
Technical Information and Editorial Services Branch
4770 Buford Highway N.E.
Atlanta, GA 30341

Phone: 770-488-5080
Fax: 770-488-5969
Email: ccdinfo@cdc.gov.
Web site: http://www.cdc.gov/nccdphp/

National Heart, Lung, and Blood Institute
P.O. Box 30105
Bethesda, MD 20824-0105
Phone: 301-592-8573
Fax: 301-592-8563
Email: nhlbiinfo@rover.nhlbi.nih.gov
Web site: http://www.nhlbi.nih.gov

National Institute for Fitness and Sport
250 N. University Boulevard
Indianapolis, IN 46202
Phone: 317-274-3432
Fax: 317-274-7408
Web site: http://www.nifs.org/

National Osteoporosis Foundation
1232 22nd Street N.W.
Washington, D.C. 20037-1292
Phone: 202-223-2226
Email: nof@nof.org
Web site: http://www.nof.org

National Wellness Institute
1300 College Court
P.O. Box 827
Stevens Point, WI 54481
Phone: 715-342 2969
          800-243-8694
Fax: 715-342-2979
Email: nwi@nationalwellness.org
Web site: http://www.nationalwellness.org

Office of Minority Health Resource Center
P.O. Box 37337
Washington, DC 20013-7337
Phone: 800-444-6472
Fax: Fax: 301-251-2160
Email: info@omhrc.gov
Web site: http://www.omhrc.gov

President's Council on Physical Fitness and Sports
Hubert H. Humphrey Bldg., Room 738H
200 Independence Avenue SW
Washington, DC 20201

Phone: 202-690-9000
Fax: 202-690-5211
Web site: http://www.fitness.gov

Road Runners Club of America
510 North Washington Street
Alexandria, Virginia 22314
Phone: 703-836-0558
Fax: 703-836-4430
Email: office@rrca.org
Web site: http://www.rrca.org

Shape Up America!
15757 Crabbs Branch Way
Rockville, MD 20855
Phone: 301-258-0540
Fax: 301-258-0541
Email: info@shapeup.org
Web site: http://www.shapeup.org

U.S. Public Health Services Office on Women's Health
8550 Arlington Blvd., Suite 300
Fairfax, VA 22031
Phone: 800-994-9662
Web site: http://www.4women.gov

Wellness Councils of America
9802 Nicholas St., Suite 315
Omaha, NE 68114
Phone: 402-827-3590
Fax: 402-827-3594
Email: wellworkplace@welcoa.org
Web site: http://www.welcoa.org

YMCA of USA
101 North Wacker Drive
Chicago, IL 60606
Phone: 312-977-0031
Web site: http://www.ymca.net

NUTRITION ORGANIZATIONS

American Dietetic Association
120 South Riverside Plaza, Suite 2000
Chicago, IL 60606-6995
Phone: 312-899-0040
              800-877-1600
Fax: 312-899-1973
Web site: http://www.eatright.org

Gatorade Sports Science Institute
617 West Main Street
Barrington, IL 60010
Phone: 312-329-7650
            800-616-4774
Email: gssi@gssiweb.com
Web site: http://www.gssiweb.com

International Food Information Council
1100 Connecticut Ave. NW, Suite 430
Washington, DC 20036
Phone: 202-296-6540
Fax: 202-296-6547
Email: foodinfo@ific.org
Web site: http://ific.org/

National Cattlemen's Beef Association
9110 East Nichols Ave #300
Centennial, CO 80112
Phone: 303-694-0305
Fax: 303-694-2851
Web site: http://www.beef.org

National Dairy Council
10255 West Higgins Road, Suite 900
Rosemont, IL 60018-5616
Phone: 847-803-2000
Fax: 847-803-2000
Email: ndc@dairyinformation.com
Web site: http://www.nationaldairycouncil.org

Society for Nutrition Education
9202 N. Meridian, Suite 200
Indianapolis, IN 46260
Phone: 317-571-5618
            800-235-6690
Fax: 317-571-5603
Email: info@sne.org
Web site: http://sne.org/

OLDER ADULTS ORGANIZATIONS

Administration on Aging
One Massachusetts Avenue
Washington, DC 20201
Phone: 202-619-0724
Email: AoAInfo@aoa.gov
Web site: http://www.aoa.gov

American Association of Retired Persons (AARP)
601 E Street NW
Washington, DC 20049
Phone: 800-424-3410
Web site: http://www.aarp.org

American Senior Fitness Association
P.O. Box 2575
New Smyrna Beach, FL 32170
Phone: 386-423-6634
         800-243-1478
Fax: 386-427-0613
Email: sfa@seniorfitness.net
Web site: http://www.seniorfitness.net/

Fitness Educators of Older Adults Association (FEOAA)
759 Chopin Drive
Sunnyvale, CA 94087
Phone: 408-450-1224
Web site: http://www.fitnesseducators.com

National Council on Aging
300 D Street, SW, Suite 801
Washington, D.C. 20024
Phone: 202-479-1200
Fax: 202-479-0735
Email: info@ncoa.org
Web site: http://www.ncoa.org

National Senior Games Association
P.O. Box 82059
Baton Rouge, LA 70884-2059
Phone: 225-379-7337
Fax: 225-379-7343
Web site: http://www.nationalseniorgames.net

RECREATION/ LEISURE ORGANIZATIONS

American Association for Leisure and Recreation
1900 Association Drive
Reston, VA 20191
Phone: 800-213-7193, Ext. 472
Web site: http://www.aahperd.org/aalr

American Camping Association
Bradford Woods
5000 State Road 67 North
Martinsville, IN 46151

Phone: 765-342-8456
Fax: 765-342-2065
Web site: http://www.acacamps.org

American Canoe Association
7432 Alban Station Blvd., Suite B232
Springfield, VA 22150
Phone: 703-451-0141
Fax: 703-451-2245
Email: aca@acanet.org
Web site: http://www.acanet.org

American Volkssport Association
1001 Pat Booker Road, Suite 101
Universal City, TX 78148
Phone: 210-659-2112
           800-830-WALK
Fax: 210-659-1212
Email: avahq@ava.org
Web site: http://www.ava.org

Family Campers and RVers
4804 Transit Road, Building 2
Depew, NY 14043
Phone: 716-668-6242
           800-245-9755
Fax: 716-668-6242
Email: office@fcrv.org
Web site: http://www.fcrv.org

National Recreation and Parks Association (NRPA)
22377 Belmont Ridge Road
Ashburn, VA 20148-4501
Phone: 703-858-0784
Fax: 703-858-0794
Email: info@nrpa.org
Web site: http://www.nrpa.org

SPORT ORGANIZATIONS

Amateur Athletic Union of the United States, Inc.
P.O. Box 22409
Lake Buena Vista, FL 32830
Phone: 407-934-7200
Fax: 407-945-7242
Web site: http://www.aausports.org

Amateur Softball Association
2801 Northeast 50th Street
Oklahoma City, OK 73111-7203

Phone: 405-424-5266
Fax: 405-424-3855
Email: Info@softball.org
Web site: http://www.softball.org

American Osteopathic Academy of Sports Medicine
7600 Terrace Avenue, Suite 203
Middleton, WI 53562
Phone: 608-831-4400
Fax: 608-831-5185
Email: info@aoasm.org
Web site: http://www.aoasm.org/

American Running and Fitness Association
4405 East West Highway, Suite 405
Bethesda, MD 20814
Phone: 800-776-ARFA
Fax: 301-913-9520
Email: arfarun@aol.com
Web site: http://www.arfa.org

American Youth Soccer Organization
12501 S. Isis Ave.
Hawthorne, CA 90250
Phone: 800-872-2796
Web site: http://www.soccer.org

Disabled Sports USA
451 Hungerford Drive, Suite 100
Rockville, MD 20850
Phone: 301-217-0960
Fax: 301-217-0968
Email: information@dsusa.org
Web site: http://www.dsusa.org

Dwarf Athletic Association of America
418 Willow Way
Lewisville TX 75077
Phone: 972-317-8299
Fax: 972-317-0184
Email: daaa@flash.net
Web site: http://www.daaa.org

International Health Racquet & Sportsclub Association (IHRSA)
263 Summer Street
Boston, MA 02210
Phone: 617-951-0055
          800-228-4772
Fax: 617-951-0056

Email: info@ihrsa.org
Web site: http://www.ihrsa.org

Jazzercise
2460 Impala Drive
Carlsbad, CA 92008
Phone: 760- 476-1750
Email: Jazzinc@jazzercise.com
Web site: http://www.jazzercise.com

National Archery Association
One Olympic Plaza
Colorado Springs, CO 80909
Phone: 719-866-4576
Fax: 719-866-4733
Email: info@usarchery.org
Web site: http://www.USArchery.org

National Association of Girls and Women in Sports
1900 Association Drive
Reston, VA 20191
Phone: 800-213-7193, Ext. 453
Web site: http://www.aahperd.org/nagws/

National Association of Intercollegiate Athletics (NAIA)
23500 W. 105th Street
PO Box 1325
Olathe, KS 66051-1325
Phone: 913-791-0044
Fax: 913-791-9555
Web site: http://www.naia.org

National Athletic Trainers Association
2952 Stemmons Freeway
Dallas, TX 75247-6916
Phone: 214-637-6282
Fax: 214-637-2206
Web site: http://www.nata.org

National Center for Bicycling and Walking
1506 21st Street NW, Suite 200
Washington, DC 20036
Phone: 202-463-6622
Fax: 202-463-6625
Email: info@bikewalk.org
Web site: http://www.bikewalk.org

National Collegiate Athletic Association
700 W. Washington Street
P.O. Box 6222

Indianapolis, Indiana 46206-6222
Phone: 317-917-6222
Fax: 317-917-6888
Web site: http://www.ncaa.org

National Congress of State Games
State Games of America
290 Roberts Street
East Hartford, CT 06108
Phone: 860-528-4588
Fax: 860-291-8032
Email: info@nutmegstategames.org
Web site: http://www.stategames.org/sgoa/info.html

National Field Archery Association
31407 Outer I-10
Redlands, CA 92373
Phone: 800-811-2331
Fax: 909-794-8512
Web site: http://www.nfaa-archery.org

National Sporting Goods Association
1601 Feehanville Drive, Suite 300
Mt. Prospect, IL 60056
Phone: 847-296-6742
         800/815-5422
Fax: 847-391-9827
Email: info@nsga.org
Web site: http://www.nsga.org

National Strength and Conditioning Association
1955 North Union Blvd.
Colorado Springs, CO 80909
Phone: 719-632-6722
         800-815-6826
Fax: 719-632-6367
Email: nsca@usa.net
Web site: http://www.nsca-lift.org

Special Olympics
1325 G Street, Suite 500
Washington, DC 20005
Phone: 202-628-3630
Fax: 202-824-0200
Email: info@specialolympics.org
Web site: http://www.specialolympics.org

United States Canoe Association, Inc.
606 Ross Street
Middletown, OH 45044-5062

Fax: 717-235-4183
Email: uscamack@aol.com
Web site: http://www.uscanoe.com

United States Field Hockey Association
One Olympic Plaza
Colorado Springs, CO 80909
Phone: 719-866-4567
Fax: 719-632-0979
Email: usfha@usfieldhockey.com
Web site: http://www.usfieldhockey.com

United States Figure Skating Association
20 First Street
Colorado Springs, CO 80906
Phone: 719-635-5200
Fax: 719-635-9548
Email: usfsa@usfsa.org
Web site: http://www.usfsa.org

United States Judo, Inc.
One Olympic Plaza, Suite 202
Colorado Springs, CO 80909
Phone: 719-866-4730
Fax: 719-866-4733
Web site: http://www.usjudo.org

United States Luge Association
35 Church Street
Lake Placid, NY 12946
Phone: 518-523-2071
Fax: 518-523-4106
Email: info@usaluge.org
Web site: http://www.usaluge.org

United States Olympic Committee
One Olympic Plaza
Colorado Springs, CO 80909
Phone: 719-866-4500
Fax: 719-866-4654
Email: media@usoc.org
Web site: http://www.olympic-usa.org

United States Synchronized Swimming
Pan Am Plaza
201 S. Capitol Avenue, Suite 901
Indianapolis, IN 46225
Phone: 317-237-5700
Fax: 317-237-5705

Web site: http://www.usasynchro.org

United States Taekwondo Union
One Olympic Plaza, Suite 104C
Colorado Springs, CO 80909
Phone: 719-866-4632
Fax: 719-866-4642
Web site: http://www.ustu.com

U.S. Association for Blind Athletes
33 North Institute
Colorado Springs, CO 80903
Phone: 719-630-0422
Fax: 719-630-0616
Email: usaba@usa.net
Web site: http://www.usaba.org

U.S. Biathlon
29 Ethan Allen Avenue
Colchester, VT 05446
Phone: 802-654-7833
               800-242-8456
Fax: 802-654-7830
Email: USBiathlon@aol.com
Web site: http://www.usbiathlon.org

U.S. Bobsled and Skeleton Federation
421 Old Military Road
Lake Placid, NY 12946
Phone: 518-523-1842
Fax: 518-523-9491
Email: info@usabobsled.org
Web site: http:// http://www.usbsf.com/index.htm

U.S. Diving, Inc.
201 South Capitol Ave., Suite 430
Indianapolis, IN 46225
Phone: 317-237-5252
Fax: 317-237-5257
Email: usdiving@usdiving.org
Web site: http://www.usdiving.org

U.S. Fencing
One Olympic Plaza, Suite 405
Colorado Springs, CO 80909
Phone: 719-866-4511
Fax: 719-632-5737
Email: info@usfencing.org
Web site: http://www.usfencing.org

U.S. Orienteering Federation
P.O. Box 1444
Forest Park, GA 30298
Phone: 404-363-2110
Fax: 404-363-2110
Web site: http://www.us.orienteering.org

U.S. Racquetball
1685 West Uintah Street
Colorado Springs, CO 80904
Phone: 719-635-5396
Fax: 719-635-0685
Email: racquetball@usra.org
Web site: http://www.usra.org

U.S. Rowing
201 South Capitol Avenue, Suite 400
Indianapolis, IN 46225
Phone: 800-314-4769
Fax: 317-237-5646
Email: members@USRowing.org

U.S. Sailing Association
15 Maritime Drive
Portsmouth, RI 02871
Phone: 401-683-0800
Fax: 401-683-0840
Email: info@ussailing.org
Web site: http://www.ussailing.org

U.S. Ski & Snowboard Association
Box 100
1500 Kearns Boulevard
Park City, UT 84060
Phone: 435-649-9090
Fax: 435-649-3613
Email: special2@ussa.org
Web site: http://www.usskiteam.com

U.S. Speedskating
P.O. Box 450639
Westlake, OH 44145
Phone: 440-899-0128
Fax: 440-899-0109
Web site: http://www.usspeedskating.org

U.S. Squash Racquets Association
P.O. Box 1216
Bala Cynwyd, PA 18004

Phone: 610-667-4006
Fax: 610-667-6539
Email: office@us-squash.org
Web site: http://www.us-squash.org/squash/ussra/

U.S. Water Polo, Inc.
1685 West Uintah
Colorado Springs, CO 80904-2921
Phone: 719-634-0699
Fax: 719-634-0866
Email: uswpoffice@uswp.org
Web site: http://www.usawaterpolo.com/

U.S. Modern Pentathlon Association
5415 Bandera Road, Suite 512
San Antonio, Texas 78238
Phone: 210-229-2004
Fax: 210-647-7194
Email: usmpa@texas.net
Web site: http://usmpa.home.texas.net

USA Badminton
One Olympic Plaza
Colorado Springs, CO 80909
Phone: 719-866-4808
Fax: 719-866-4507
Email: usab@usabadminton.org
Web site: http://www.usabadminton.org

USA Baseball
P.O. Box 1131
Durham, NC 27702
Phone: 919-474-8721
Fax: 919-474-8822
Email: info@usabaseball.com
Web site: http://www.usabaseball.com

USA Basketball
5465 Mark Dabling Boulevard
Colorado Springs, CO 80918
Phone: 719-590-4800
Fax: 719-590-4811
Email: fanmail@usabasketball.com
Web site: http://www.usabasketball.com

USA Boxing
One Olympic Plaza
Colorado Springs, CO 80909
Phone: 719-866-4506

Fax: 719-632-3426
Email: jgoldsticker@usaboxing.org
Web site: http://www.usaboxing.org

USA Bowling
5301 South 76th Street
Greendale, WI 53129-0500
Phone: 414-421-9008
              800-514-2695
Fax: 414-421-1301
Email: info@usabowling.org
Web site: http://www.bowl.com

USA Cycling
One Olympic Plaza
Colorado Springs, CO 80909
Phone: 719-866-4581
Fax: 719-866-4628
Email: membership@usacycling.org
Web site: http://www.usacycling.org

USA Gymnastics
Pan American Plaza, Suite 300
201 South Capitol Avenue
Indianapolis, IN 46225
Phone: 317-237-5050
Fax: 317-237-5069
Web site: http://www.usa-gymnastics.org

USA Hockey, Inc.
1775 Bob Johnson Drive
Colorado Springs, CO 80906
Phone: 719-576-8724
Fax: 719-538-1160
Email: usah@usahockey.org
Web site: http://www.usahockey.com

USA Roller Sports
4730 South Street
Lincoln, NE 68506
Phone: 402-483-7551
Fax: 402-483-1465
Web site: http://www.usarollersports.com

USA Shooting
One Olympic Plaza
Colorado Springs, CO 80909
Phone: 719-866-4670

Email: Admin.Info@usashooting.org
Web site: http://www.usashooting.org

USA Swimming
One Olympic Plaza
Colorado Springs, CO 80909
Phone: 719-866-4578
Web site: http://www.usa-swimming.org

USA Table Tennis Association
One Olympic Plaza
Colorado Springs, CO 80909
Phone: 719-866-4583
Fax: 719-632-6071
Email: usatt@usatt.org
Web site: http://www.usatt.org

USA Team Handball
One Olympic Plaza
Colorado Springs, CO 80909
Phone: 719-866-4036
Fax: 719-866-4055
Email: info@usateamhandball.org
Web site: http://www.usateamhandball.org

USA Track and Field
1 RCA Dome, Suite 140
Indianapolis, IN 46225
Phone: 317-261-0500
Fax: 317-261-0481
Web site: http://www.usatf.org

USA Volleyball
715 S. Circle Dr.
Colorado Springs, CO 80910
Phone: 719-228-6800
              888-786-5539 (Information Line)
Fax: 719 228-6899
Web site: http://www.usavolleyball.org

USA Weightlifting, Inc.
One Olympic Plaza
Colorado Springs, Co 80909
Phone: 719-866-4508
Fax: 719-866-4741
Email: usaw@usaweightlifting.org
Web site: http://www.usaweightlifting.org

USA Wrestling
6155 Lehman Drive
Colorado Springs, CO 80918
Phone: 719-598-8181
Fax: 719-598-9440
Web site: http://www.usawrestling.org

Wheelchair Sports, USA
3595 East Fountain Boulevard, Suite L-1
Colorado Springs, CO 80910
Phone: 719-574-1150
Fax: 719-574-9840
Email: wsusa@aol.com
Web site: http://www.wsusa.org

Women's Sports Foundation
Eisenhower Park, East Meadows
New York, NY 11554
Phone: 800-227-3988
Fax: 516-542-4716
Email: Wosport@aol.com
Web site: http://www.womenssportsfoundation.org

YOUTH ORGANIZATIONS

National Youth Sports Safety Foundation, Inc
One Beacon Street, Suite 3333
Boston, Massachusetts 02108
Phone: 617-277-1171
Fax: 617-722-9999
E Mail: NYSSF@aol.com
Web site: http://www.nyssf.org

YWCA of the U.S.A.
1015 18th Street, NW, Suite 700
Washington, DC 20036
Phone: 202-467-0801
               800-YWCA-US1
Fax: 202-467-0802
Web site: http://www.ywca.org

APPENDIX B

Professional Journals Relating to Physical Education and Sport

Each entry includes the journal title, aim, publisher, address, and telephone, when available.

Academy Papers
Papers presented at annual meetings of the academy
American Academy of Kinesiology and Physical Education
Human Kinetics Publishers, Inc.
Box 5076
Champaign, IL 61825-5076
800-747-4457

Adapted Physical Activity Quarterly
Teaching/research consisting of case studies
Human Kinetics Publishers, Inc.
Box 5076
Champaign, IL 61825-5076
800-747-4457

American Fitness
Materials concerning aerobics, health, and fitness
Aerobics and Fitness Association of America
15250 Ventura Boulevard,
Suite 200
Sherman Oaks, CA 91403
800-446-2322

American Health
Research magazine for health, fitness, and medicine
American Health
19 W. 22nd Street
New York, NY 10010
212-366-8900

American Journal of Public Health
Diverse types of articles for professionals in health
American Public Health Association
1015 Fifteenth Street NW, Suite 300
Washington, DC 20005
202-789-5600

American Journal of Sports Medicine
Articles related to sports medicine
American Orthopaedic Society for Sports Medicine
230 Calvary Street
Waltham, MA 02154
617-736-0707

Athletic Administration
Administrative materials and articles
National Association of Collegiate Directors of Athletics
P.O. Box 16428
Cleveland, OH 44116
216-892-4000

Athletic Business
Information about facilities, management, and financing
1846 Hoffman Street
Madison, WI 53704
608-249-0186

CAHPER Journal
Information on all aspects of HPERD profession
Canadian Association for HPER
Place R. Tait McKenzie
1600 James Naismith Drive
Gloucester Ont. 5 N4 Canada
613-748-5622

Clinical Journal of Sports Medicine
Research articles, case reports, and new procedures in sports medicine
Canadian Academy of Sports Medicine
Lippincott Williams & Wilkins
530 Walnut Street
Philadelphia, PA 19016
Phone: 215-521-8300

Dance Magazine
Articles focus on dance performance
33 West 60th Street
New York, NY 10023-7990
212-245-9050

Health Education Quarterly
Articles promoting health , practice of medicine, and research
Society for Public Health Education
John Wiley and Sons, Inc.
605 3rd Avenue
New York, NY 10158
212-850-6000

IDEA Personal Trainer
Articles concerning fitness education
International Assoc. of Fitness Professionals
6190 Cornerstone Court East, Suite 204
San Diego, CA 92121-3773
800-747-4457

International Journal of Sport Biomechanics
Articles on theory and research
Human Kinetics Publishers, Inc.
Box 5076
Champaign, IL 61825-5076

Interscholastic Athletic Administration
High school athletic programs
National Federation of State High School Associations
11724 NW Plaza Circle
P.O. Box 20626
Kansas City, MO 64195-0626
816-464-5400

Journal of Applied Sport Psychology
Articles concerning sport psychology
Association for the Advancement of Applied Sport Psychology
Bowling Green State University
Eppler Center
Bowling Green, OH 43403
419-372-7233

Journal of Athletic Training
Articles about athletic training
National Athletic Trainers' Association
2952 Stemmons Freeway, Suite 200
Dallas, TX 75247-6103
800-879-6282

Journal of Health Education
Articles on health education
American Association for Health Education of the American
Alliance for Health, Physical Education, Recreation and Dance
1900 Association Drive
Reston, VA 22091-1599
800-213-7193

Journal of the International Council for Health,
Physical Education and Recreation, Dance and Sport
Articles with emphasis on research and teaching
American Alliance for Health, Physical Education, Recreation and Dance
1900 Association Drive
Reston, VA 22091-1599
800-213-7193

Journal of Leisure Research
Research and articles in leisure
National Recreation and Park Association
2755 S. Quincy Street, Suite 300

Arlington, VA 22206-2204
703-820-4940

Journal of Motor Behavior
Articles concerning human movement
Heldref Publications
1319 Eighteenth Street NW
Washington, DC 20036-1802
202-296-5149

Journal of the Philosophy of Sport
Philosophical articles about sports
Philosophic Society for the Study of Sport
Human Kinetics Publishers, Inc.
Box 5076
Champaign, IL 61825-5076
800-747-4457

Journal of Physical Education, Recreation and Dance
Practical and informational articles concerning health, physical
education, recreation, dance and sports
American Alliance for Health, Physical Education,
Recreation and Dance
1900 Association Drive
Reston, VA 22091-1599
800-213-7193

Journal of School Health
Articles on education and the promotion of health
American School Health Association
P.O. Box 708
Kent, OH 44240
216-678-1601

Journal of Sport and Exercise Psychology
Research articles
Human Kinetics Publishers, Inc.
Box 5076
Champaign, IL 61825-5076
800-747-4457

Journal of Sport History
Research concerning sport history
North American Society for Sport History
101 White Building
Pennsylvania State University
University Park, PA 16802-3903
814-238-1288

Journal of Sport Management
Practical and theoretical articles
North American Society for Sport Management
Human Kinetics Publishers, Inc.
Box 5076
Champaign, IL 61825-5076
800-747-4457

Journal of Strength and Conditioning Research
Research relating to the conditioning of athletes
National Strength and Conditioning Association
Human Kinetics Publishers, Inc.
Box 5076
Champaign, IL 61825-5076
800-747-4457

Journal of Teaching in Physical Education
Research in teacher education
Human Kinetics Publishers, Inc.
Box 5076
Champaign, IL 61825-5076
800-747-4457

Medicine and Science in Sports and Exercise
Research concerning the scientific aspects of sports and exercise
American College of Sports Medicine
Box 1440
Indianapolis, IN 46206-1440
317-637-9200

National Coach: The Voice of High School Coaches in America
Articles on aspects of coaching
National High School Athletic Coaches Association
P.O. Box 5020
Winter Park, FL 32793-5020
407-679-1414

NIRSA Journal
Articles for college intramural personnel
National Intramural-Recreational Sports Association
850 SW 15th Street
Corvallis, OR 97333
507-737-2088

Parks and Recreation
Research articles in leisure services
National Recreation and Park Association
2775 S. Quincy Street,

Suite 300
Arlington, VA 22206-2204
703-820-2162

Perceptual and Motor Skills
Articles relating to perception and motor skills
Psychological Reports
Box 9229
Missoula, MT 59807-9229
406-728-1710

The Physical Educator
Articles concerning physical education and other related fields
Phi Epsilon Kappa
910 W. New York Street
Indianapolis, IN 46202
317-637-8431

Physical Therapy
Research and practical articles for physical therapists
American Physical Therapy Association
1111 North Fairfax Street
Alexandria, VA 22314
703-684-2782

The Physician and Sportsmedicine
Practical and theoretical articles concerning
the medical aspects of exercise, fitness, and sports
McGraw-Hill Healthcare Group
4530 W. 77th Street
Minneapolis, MN 55435
612-835-3222

Quest
Articles concerning important issues in higher education
National Association for Physical Education in Higher Education
Human Kinetics Publishers, Inc.
Box 5076
Champaign, IL 61825-5076
800-747-4457

Research Quarterly for Exercise and Sport
Scholarly articles
American Alliance for Health, Physical Education, Recreation and
Dance
1900 Association Drive
Reston, VA 22091-1599
800-213-7193

Scholastic Coach
Practical articles for coaches
Scholastic, Inc.
555 Broadway
New York, NY 10003
213-343-6100

Sociology of Sport Journal
Practical and theoretical papers
North American Society for the Sociology of Sport
Human Kinetics Publishers, Inc.
Box 5076
Champaign, IL 61825-5076
800-747-4457

The Sport Psychologist
Articles on the psychological aspects of sport and physical activity
Human Kinetics Publishers, Inc.
Box 5076
Champaign, IL 61825-5076
800-747-4457

Sport Science Review
Articles concerning scientific studies in physical education and sport
International Council of Sport Science and Physical Education
Human Kinetics Publishers, Inc.
Box 5076
Champaign, IL 61825-5076
800-747-4457

Strategies: A Journal for Sport and Physical Educators
Articles to improve teaching and coaching
National Association for Girls and Women in Sport and
National Association for Sport and Physical Education of
the American Alliance for Health, Physical Education,
Recreation and Dance
1900 Association Drive
Reston, VA 22091-1599
800-213-7193

Strength and Conditioning
Practical and theoretical articles on strength and conditioning
National Strength and Conditioning Association
Human Kinetics Publishers, Inc.
Box 5076
Champaign, IL 61825-5076
800-747-4457

Therapeutic Recreation Journal
Practical use articles
National Recreation and Park Association
2775 S. Quincy Street,
Suite 300
Arlington, VA 22206-2204
703-820-2162

Women's Sports and Fitness
Practical articles on women and sports
2025 Pearl Street
Boulder, CO 80302
303-440-5111

Youth Sports Coach
Practical articles concerning coaches of youth sports
National Youth Sports Coaches Association
2050 Vista Parkway
West Palm Beach, FL 33411-2718
800-729-2057

Answers to Multiple Choice Questions

Chapter 1
1 b, 2 d, 3 a, 4 d, 5 c, 6 a, 7 b, 8 d, 9 c, 10 c

Chapter 2
1 d, 2 b, 3 a, 4 e, 5 a, 6 b, 7 d, 8 c, 9 d, 10 d

Chapter 3
1 a, 2 a, 3 d, 4 d, 5 a, 6 d, 7 b, 8 e, 9 a, 10 e

Chapter 4
1 c, 2 e, 3 c, 4 a, 5 b, 6 b, 7 e, 8 c, 9 c, 10 e

Chapter 5
1 a, 2 e, 3 e, 4 e, 5 c, 6 c, 7 a, 8 c, 9 a, 10 c

Chapter 6
1 c, 2 b, 3 c, 4 a, 5 e, 6 b, 7 c, 8 b, 9 e, 10 c

Chapter 7
1 d, 2 e, 3 b, 4 b, 5 d, 6 e, 7 a, 8 b, 9 b, 10 b

Chapter 8
1 a, 2 d, 3 a, 4 e, 5 c, 6 a, 7 a, 8 d, 9 b, 10 e

Chapter 9
1 b, 2 c, 3 d, 4 c, 5 c, 6 b, 7 d, 8 b, 9 d, 10 a

Chapter 10
1 a, 2 b, 3 c, 4 b, 5 d, 6 c, 7 b, 8 a, 9 c, 10 d

Glossary

academic discipline The body of knowledge that constitutes a subject area; physical education, social studies, or mathematics, for example.

adapted physical education Also called "special physical education"; strives to provide equal opportunities for everyone—including those with disabilities—to participate in physical activity and sport.

adventure education A curriculum area that includes outdoor activities, such as backpacking, orienteering, camping, canoeing, and rock climbing, as well as controlled risk-taking activities on low and high ropes courses to develop trust, confidence, and cooperation.

Aerobics Kenneth Cooper's seminal work (1968) that popularized cardiorespiratory fitness in America by simplifying technical physiological measurements of the body's ability to use oxygen into easily understood concepts.

aesthetics The branch of philosophy concerned with the appreciation of beauty, taste, and the quality of life.

affective goals Physical education objectives that promote an appreciation for and positive attitude toward physical activity through pleasurable and meaningful experiences.

allied areas of specialization Initially, career options for physical education students who witnessed a great decline of teaching positions during the 1970s. Now these specializations, such as athletic training and sports management, have become degree programs that attract their own pool of students.

allied fields The fields of health, recreation, dance, athletic training, and sports management that share some purposes, programs, and professional activities with physical education and sport.

anthropometric measurement Bodily measurements (height, weight, arm, chest, waist girth, and the like) taken by Edward Hitchcock, Dudley Sargent, Delphine Hanna, and other early physical educators to develop norms and classify college students.

arête Greek conception of excellence in all facets of life: physical, intellectual, and spiritual. An ideal that Greeks strove for, but few ever reached it.

aritomism A philosophical approach that seeks absolute, unchanging truths that are universal for all people at all times.

asceticism A belief and practice in which spiritual development is emphasized over bodily needs as a path to salvation; involves suppression of animal instincts.

Association for the Advancement of Physical Education (AAPE) Original name of AAHPERD, founded in 1885 as an outgrowth of a meeting of physicians, gymnasium directors, and others involved in the instruction of physical activity.

Association for Intercollegiate Athletics for Women (AIAW) An organization formed from CIAW in 1971 to bring more direction and governance to women's sports.

athletic training Deals with the prevention, treatment, and rehabilitation of injuries that result from physical activity and athletic competition.

"athletics are educational" doctrine Belief that athletics had redeeming educational values; enabled school administrators and educators to justify the existence of interscholastic athletics.

axiology The branch of philosophy concerned with values.

Battle of the Systems Debate between the proponents of German and Swedish gymnastics over the merits of each system.

biomechanics The study and analysis of the mechanics of human movement, with efficient movement as a goal.

block scheduling Method of scheduling in which, classes meet for longer periods of times (usually twice the length or a traditional period or ninety minutes); there are fewer periods each day and usually fewer days of instruction. In block scheduling, the instruction is more concentrated.

Boston Conference on Physical Training Conference in 1889 financed by Mary Hemenway to provide an open forum for the discussion of German, Swedish, and other gymnastics systems in use. It was chaired by U.S. Commissioner of Education William T. Harris and attracted more than 2,000 people.

Boston Normal School of Gymnastics Founded and financed by Mary Hemenway and headed by Amy Morris Homans for the preparation of young women to teach Swedish gymnastics. It was an outgrowth of the Swedish-German gymnastics debate.

brain-based instruction Teaching and curriculum based on the way the brain works. The physical education classroom is highly brain-compatible: It offers the stimulation, repetition, and novelty that enhance learning.

Campus Martius Parade ground where youth and men trained and developed their military skills.

cathedral schools Established at cathedrals in medieval cities to train clerics for each bishopric or diocese; they accepted lay students.

certification A statement or document indicating the fulfillment of requirements that grants one permission to practice or carry out occupational duties in a specific field.

Christian physiology An early-nineteenth-century belief and moral standard promoted by Sylvester Graham and William Alcott; it viewed all bodily ailments as gastrointestinal, caused by improper diet and imbibing alcohol. An ailing body, in turn, damaged the soul.

Circus Maximus Largest arena in Rome, where chariot races were held before an estimated 150,000 to 250,000 spectators.

cognitive goals Physical education objectives that advocate challenging physical activities involving problem solving, cooperative ventures, or individual self-expression to stimulate thought processes.

collaboration Process in which teachers from each discipline work together to identify and discuss problems that inhibit learning. Collaboration can also occur between the school and two or more entities in the community.

Colosseum Prominent arena in Rome where gladiatorial combat was held.

Commission for Intercollegiate Athletics for Women (CIAW) A subunit of the Division of Girls and Women's Sports (DGWS) within AAHPER that was organized in 1966 to promote varsity athletics for girls and women.

Committee on Women's Athletics (CWA) A committee within the American Physical Education Association (APEA) organized in 1917 by female physical educators to maintain control of women's athletics.

core content knowledge A set of crucial (or core) courses that represent the body of knowledge of a given discipline. In physical education, core content courses are anatomy and physiology, physiology of exercise, biomechanics, motor behavior, psychology and sociology of sport, history and philosophy of the discipline and profession.

court ball Rigorous ball game played by Aztec and Mayan Indians on an I-shaped court. Objective was to propel a softball-sized rubber ball through a ring without using the hands or feet.

crown games Panhellenic athletic competitions held during non-Olympic years at Delphi, Corinth, and Nemea.

Cult of True Womanhood Nineteenth-century conception of the traits and characteristics an upper- and middle-class woman should possess—piety, purity, submissiveness, and domesticity.

culture The sum total of ways of living that have evolved for a group of human beings and have been transmitted from one group to another. A collection of individual life experiences; includes ethnicity, religion, gender, interests, activities, abilities, social class, professions, customs, and lifestyles.

discipline The body of knowledge that constitutes physical education.

distance learning Education delivered via video or computer to students who are not in the same location as the teacher—in fact, who are anywhere in the world.

diversity Heterogeneous mix of religion, ethnicity, gender, and sexual orientation in groups of people in various environments; for our purposes, in the educational setting; the. state of having varied, and unlike, qualities or elements.

dualism A belief in the separation of mind and body.

eclecticism In terms of personal philosophy, the acceptance of ideas, thoughts, beliefs, and practices from two or more philosophical approaches.

electronic mailing lists Private discussion groups that provide a forum, via the Internet, for people with common interests to pose questions, engage in discussions, and share their views. Messages are exchanged via email; participation requires "subscription," which may be limited and require approval by a "moderator." Some electronic mailing lists are open to anyone.

email A quick method of sending and receiving messages via computer and an Internet connection.

Enlightenment Eighteenth-century movement growing out of Renaissance; it emphasized inalienable rights of humankind and its quest to master the environment through critical analysis and scientific investigation.

epistemology The branch of philosophy that deals with the acquisition of knowledge.

Equity in Athletics Disclosure Act of 1996 Federal legislation that requires colleges and universities to meet the proportionality test in which the proportion of athletes in the underrepresented gender must be within 5 percent of the underrepresented gender's enrollment.

essentialism A belief in a basic core of knowledge, skills, and values that should be instilled in all learners.

ethics A dimension of axiology that deals with moral judgments, questions of how individuals treat each other and themselves.

ethnic Pertaining to groups of people categorized according to shared national, religious, linguistic, or cultural origin or background.

exercise gerontology The combination of exercise physiology principles with theories of aging in order to help older adults maintain their independence and a decent quality of life.

exercise physiology The study of the human body's response to exercise and physical activity.

exercise psychology The study of psychology as it relates to exercise and motivation to continue to exercise on a regular basis.

existentialism A modern philosophy based on the absurdity of life and knowing the inner self. It predicates freedom of choice and the need to accept responsibility for one's own life in order to become the best one can become.

Festival of Sed Egyptian festival during which pharaohs ran on semicircular tracks to demonstrate their physical attributes and symbolically to renew their strength.

feudalism A system of political organization in which the lord or king held all land in fee; vassals (subordinates) administered and paid homage to the lord with foods, clothing, and other goods; in return, vassals and their tenants (serfs) received protection through the lord's military legion.

fitness education Process of developing and improving health-related fitness components (cardiovascular endurance, muscular strength, muscular endurance, flexibility, and body composition).

Food Guide Pyramid An aid to following fitness guidelines; it groups foods into six categories, indicating serving sizes for each.

gladiatorial combat Fights, sometimes to the death, between two or more gladiators who were trained in the use of a variety of weapons.

gymnasia Public buildings in city-states where male Greek citizens participated in exercises, boxing, wrestling, pentathlon, and *pankration*.

Harvard Fatigue Laboratory Physiology laboratory established at Harvard in 1927 to assess performance in the workplace; during World War II it turned to investigating the limitations of physical fitness, the effects of cold and altitude on clothing and equipment, and transport of gases in the blood. It closed in 1947, but its major contribution was to provide a training ground for physiologists who would establish the field of physiology of exercise.

health-enhancing physical activity Regular physical activity that results in substantial improvements in health and well-being. Health-related fitness components include cardiovascular efficiency, muscular strength, muscular endurance, flexibility, and body composition.

health promotion An allied area of specialization whose focus is to help people attain optimal health, or wellness, through behavioral changes.

healthy life expectancy (HLE) Refers to the number of years a person is expected to live in good health. This number is obtained by subtracting ill-health years from the overall life expectancy.

Heraia Athletic competition (prenuptial rites of passage) for adolescent women held at Olympia one month before the Olympic Games.

humanism Intellectual and artistic movement that manifests a strong interest in human nature, welfare of humanity, and appreciation for joy and beauty in life; a philosophy that emphasizes the value of the human being and the power of human intelligence as well as appreciation and respect for the human body.

hypokinetic disease Lack of or too little activity; a controllable risk factor of coronary heart disease.

idealism The traditional philosophy in which only ideas are real, and the world of the material is not real.

inclusion The philosophy of merging special and general education and placing all children with disabilities in a general education setting.

individualized education program (IEP) Program that outlines the educational placements appropriate for a student with an identified disability; also identifies present levels of performance and goals for the future.

Individuals with Disabilities Education Act (IDEA) A law passed in 1990 that stated that all students with disabilities are entitled to an education in the least restrictive environment.

interactive behavior Refers to safe practices, adherence to rules and procedures, etiquette, cooperation, teamwork, ethical behavior in sports, and positive social interaction when participating in physical activity. Also includes the intrinsic value and benefits of participation in physical activity.

interactive television (ITV) Service that enables instruction to occur in two or more settings simultaneously through technology of two-way video and audio communication.

interdisciplinary unit A unit of instruction in which several curriculum areas are taught together, either in one curricular area or in cooperation with several curriculum areas.

joust Contest in which two knights tried to unseat each other from their horses.

kinesiology A multifaceted field of study in which movement or physical activity is the intellectual focus.

Kraus-Weber Test of Minimum Muscular Fitness Tests administered to American and European schoolchildren in 1953 in which 56.6 percent of the Americans and 8.2 percent of the Europeans failed. Results of this test sparked a physical fitness explosion during the 1950s.

lacrosse North American Indians played this game of dexterity in which sticks with small baskets were used to catch and propel a small ball into a small goal.

least restrictive environment Term for requirement that all students be placed in the setting that will result in the best opportunity for success and educational progress. Placements range from a special adapted physical education classroom to inclusion in the regular physical education classroom with no adaptations.

logic The branch of philosophy that involves the use of thought processes and reasoning power to reach correct conclusions.

mancalo Board game played by people of sub-Saharan Africa that involved placing objects in strategic positions to capture opponents' objects.

melee Contests in which teams of knights jousted simultaneously against each other.

metaphysics The branch of philosophy that is concerned with the nature of reality—questions about mind and body, the existence of God, and the nature of being, among others.

monastic schools Established in the monasteries to teach monks and novitiates to read scripture; they sometimes accepted lay students from privileged families.

motor behavior Broad-based term that denotes the neuromuscular basis for movement patterns in performing physical skills; it includes motor control, motor development, and motor learning.

motor control The mental processes involved in the performance of motor and physical performance skills.

motor development The growth and development of the body in relationship to the acquisition of movement skills.

motor learning Motor-skill acquisition and changes in performance of physical skills.

motor skill development Refers to the basic fundamental movement patterns that are necessary to perform a variety of physical activities. Consists of locomotor, nonlocomotor, and manipulative skills.

multiculturalism Respect for and integration of various cultures.

National Amateur Athletic Federation (NAAF) An organization founded in 1923 to challenge the Amateur Athletic Union (AAU) for control of amateur sport in America.

nationalism Loyalty and devotion to one's country; pride in one's homeland.

National Physical Education Service Supported by the Playground and Recreation Association and headed by James E. "Jimmy" Rogers, this organization emerged in 1918 to promote compulsory physical education and to assist state departments of education in the implementation of physical education programs.

naturalism The oldest philosophy, which holds that all truth and reality are found in the laws of nature and material things; it denies the supernatural.

new physical education Curriculum based on natural activities and sports and games that came into being during the Progressive era.

newsgroups Public discussion forums on specific topics, with all messages posted (as on a bulletin board) for users to view. Anyone with Internet access can read all messages and replies between the participants.

non-zero-sum competition Situation in which participants work to meet a predetermined standard or improve their own previous best performance; contrasted with traditional competition that has winners and losers.

North American turnerbund Organization of German turner societies in North America that sponsored annual festivals, turnfests, and other functions.

Olympic Games In ancient Greece, the primary festival consisting of athletic competitions held every forty-eight lunar months.

palestra Literally, a wrestling school; a place, generally private, where young Greek boys were taught the skills of wrestling by a trainer known as a *paidotribe*.

Panathenaic Festival One of the most prominent of ancient Greece's local festivals held at Athens.

pankration Athletic contest that involves elements of boxing, wrestling, and kicking. Victory requires the submission of one of the contestants.

pedagogy The study of teaching that involves the curriculum and instructional methods.

pentathlon Athletic contest in which five events are performed: foot race, discus, javelin, long jump, and wrestling. The first contestant to win three events was declared the winner.

personal philosophy The sum of one's fundamental values, beliefs, attitudes, goals, objectives, criteria, and standards; one's personal philosophy shapes one's actions.

philosophy An academic discipline; also any one of various established or traditional ways of looking at the world (such as idealism or existentialism) that have been defined and identified by those who practice the discipline, whether in the academy or not.

Physical Activity Pyramid Grouping of physical activity guidelines into five categories, with recommendations for each category.

play days Social functions in which female students from several colleges gathered for sporting and social activities. They formed composite sports teams consisting of one player from each school and played exhibition matches against one another. Afterward, the students socialized over refreshments.

praetor Political office in Rome that *aediles* sought; praetors performed judicial duties and headed the courts.

pragmatism A modern philosophy which holds that experience is the only source of truth and that what experience teaches is valuable only if it has practical applications and helps people achieve their goals.

President's Council on Youth Fitness Organized in 1956 as one reaction to the performance of American schoolchildren on the Kraus-Weber test. Today, the agency is known at the President's Council on Physical Fitness and Sports (PCPFS).

profession An occupation requiring specialized education and training; a profession usually has a set of standards for entry and a certification or licensing process.

progressive education Movement that grew out of Progressivism and led by John Dewey, G. Stanley Hall, and others; it established a child-centered curriculum based on pupils' maturation levels to facilitate learning and prepare youth to function effectively in a democratic society.

Progressivism Reform movement of the late nineteenth and early twentieth century that produced significant changes in government, agriculture, banking, business, social services, urban housing, and education.

psychomotor goals Physical education objectives that emphasize performance competencies.

realism The traditional philosophy, opposed to realism, which holds that things do exist independently of the human mind.

Reformation Religious movement in which the doctrine and practices of the Roman Catholic Church were questioned; led to establishment of Protestant denominations.

Renaissance Period in history between Middle Ages and modern period (fourteenth to seventeenth centuries) characterized by the rebirth of Greek and Roman art, literature, and ideology.

ring tourney Popular activity in Southern states in which a horse rider at full gallop attempted to insert his lance into a small suspended ring.

Round Hill School Early boarding school in Northampton, Massachusetts, designed to improve the cognitive, moral, and physical attributes of adolescent boys. Charles Beck introduced Jahn's gymnastics there, making it the first program of regular physical activity in an American curriculum.

Scholasticism Christian philosophy of the Middle Ages that stressed analysis of the Bible and other religious writings; faith was built on the revealed word of God and the wisdom of Christian thinkers.

scientization of physical education The movement of physical education toward a scientific basis with the adoption of more science-oriented courses in the curriculum, affiliation with science-based professional organizations, and modification of departments' names to include science or some variation of it.

shinny Game, similar to modern field hockey, played by North American Indians.

sport pedagogy A term with international meaning in that physical education methodologies and curriculum development are applied beyond the school setting to organizations, athletic teams, and sports clubs in the community.

sport psychology The study of psychological and behavioral issues as they relate to sport.

sports days Social functions that evolved from play days in which all female participants represented their respective schools, but participation rather than competition was emphasized.

sports management An allied specialization program that involves the business aspects of sport, especially such areas as promotion, marketing, public relations, and finance. Graduates of sports management programs work as administrators and assistant administrators for professional sports teams and leagues as well as colleges and universities.

sport sociology The study of the structure and patterns of social organizations and the dynamics of groups participating in sport.

standards Prescribed levels of performance that indicate what students should know and what they should be able to do.

Title IX of the Education Amendments Act of 1972 A law passed in 1972 that requires every educational program receiving federal assistance to provide equal opportunities and equal funding for males and females.

tournament Events in which knights maintained their military and fighting skills through jousting and melee contests.

turners German immigrants who brought to America their system of gymnastics, which they learned as members of the turnverein in Prussia and other German states.

turnverein Gymnastic clubs for German youth established by Friedrich Jahn in early nineteenth century as a reaction to Napoleon's conquests and occupation of Prussia.

Victorian era Period of history throughout most of the nineteenth century that mirrored the reign of Queen Victoria in England, 1837–1901.

virtual reality Using the computers and sensory mechanisms to create simulated, interactive three-dimensional environments.

wellness Optimal health and total well-being, generally involving physical, intellectual, social, emotional, and spiritual dimensions.

yoga In India and Asia, the practice of spiritual cleansing through meditation.

zane Statue erected at Olympia in the image of the god Zeus, to memorialize for posterity those who cheated at the Olympic Games.

zero-sum competition Traditional competitive situation in which the outcome leads to one winner and one loser.

Photo Credits

Index